A Parent's Guide to

Complementary Healthcare for Children

GW00708308

A Parent's Guide to

Complementary Healthcare for Children

PIPPA DUNCAN

NEWLEAF

First published 1997 by Newleaf

an imprint of Macmillan Publishers Ltd
25 Eccleston Place, London SW1W 9NF
and Basingstoke

Associated companies throughout the world

ISBN 0 7522 0519 6

Jacket design by Slatter-Anderson
Main cover photograph by Damian Walker
Inset photographs (top) © Tony Stone Images/Phil Borges;
bottom © Tony Stone Images/Gary Nolton
Illustrations by Cath Knox

1 3 5 7 9 8 6 4 2

A CIP catalogue entry for this book is available from the
British Library

Typeset by SX Composing DTP, Rayleigh, Essex
Printed and bound in Great Britain by
Mackays of Chatham plc, Chatham, Kent

To Alex & Jonah

Advice to the Reader

Before following any advice contained in this book, you should consult your doctor if you or your child or anyone else being treated according to or following the advice in this book suffer from any health problems or special conditions or are in any doubt as to its suitability, as it is not possible to predict an individual's reaction to a particular treatment or therapy. The author also cannot assure or be responsible for the result of any individual person's treatment or use of information given in this book, although she has taken due care to ensure that the information, advice, suggestions and opinions in this book reflect best current practice, knowledge and research in complementary medicine.

Acknowledgements

I would like to thank the following people, without whose knowledge, time and patience, this book would not be possible:

Consultant paediatrician Dr Eman Jurges of Queen Mary's University Hospital, Roehampton; naturopath Jaine Kirtley MRN RN; osteopath Mark Wilson DO MRO; acupuncturist Colin Rogers Lic Ac Cert. Ac. (Nanjing) MBAc C; homoeopath Zofia Dymitr RSHom, chairwoman of the Society of Homoeopaths; chiropractor Louise Corlet BCA; medical herbalist Linda Bostock MNIMH; hypnotherapist Mick Garrett, director of The Psycho Semantics Institute and chairman of the Association of Hypnotherapy Organizations; kinesiologist Claire Moffat ASK of the Academy of Systematic Kinesiology; reflexologist Alison Lock MAR; practitioner of traditional Chinese medicine, Helen Fielding MBAcC RCCM; aromatherapist Debbie Moore of the Shirley Price International College of Aromatherapy; Stefan Ball of the Dr Edward Bach Centre.

CONTENTS

Contents

SECTION II: THE THERAPIES

SECTION III: REMEDIES FOR THE HOME

INTRODUCTION

There are many parents who feel they would like to be able to offer their children more when it comes to their health.

Modern medicine obviously has a lot to offer and can mean the difference between life and death. But it doesn't always provide the total care that parents need, particularly for some childhood ailments. I have taken my son Jonah to the doctor for various ailments and often a prescription has been written out within minutes. I remember one time asking whether it was actually necessary for him to have antibiotics, to be told, 'Well, no not really, but it might help to get him better more quickly.' If the prescription wasn't really necessary, then I certainly didn't want to give Jonah medication he could do without. Antibiotics are precious drugs which should be saved for when really needed, not doled out for every slight infection.

But there have been times when I wasn't happy just to let Jonah 'sit it out'. I like the philosophy of complementary therapies – that they help the body to heal itself. Jonah has benefited from various therapies since he was born. When he was only three weeks old, an osteopath carried out craniosacral work to help relieve colic. The difference was amazing. A fractious, obviously uncomfortable baby was transformed into a contented child. Once, when he fell down a flight of stairs I called in the osteopath again to check he hadn't damaged his back or neck. Luckily, apart from a minor bump on the head, he was fine.

Often, as a small baby, I would massage him with aromatherapy oils blended specially for him. Not only would he lie relaxed and gurgling, but it was always a special time of closeness as I gently rubbed his tiny limbs.

Asthma and eczema run in my family, so when he seemed to have a constant cold, we visited a naturopath to try and determine any possible allergies. Switching to goats' milk and cutting out dairy products helped to reduce the amount of mucus he was producing. When he seemed particularly bad, he was also given a homoeopathic remedy to help boost his system and within days he had improved.

Having read and written on the subject, I was probably more aware than a lot of parents about which therapies may be helpful for which ailments. But for many, there are a lot of questions to be answered. Hopefully this book will go some way to helping parents and guiding them to a therapy that best suits their child.

So what are the alternatives?

What is Complementary Medicine?

Complementary medicine is not one but many therapies, which is why it can help so many different childhood ailments. Complementary therapists or practitioners do not use drugs, but treatment will depend on the type of therapy. For instance homoeopaths, herbalists and Chinese doctors use natural substances, such as herbs and vegetable matter as part of treatment, while osteopaths and chiropractors use a hands-on approach to correct musculo-skeletal-related problems. Then again, reflexologists and aromatherapists use massage and essential oils to help heal, while a naturopath may use a combination of any of these. What they all have in common is that they treat the child holistically – as a whole being. That means that not just the symptoms presented to them will be looked at, but the child as a whole will be treated. Questions such as what is their general health like, what is their diet like and how regular are their bowel movements will be asked to build up a full picture of your child's mental and emotional as well as physical wellbeing.

Even the term 'complementary medicine' can be confusing. What is the difference between it and 'alternative healthcare'? Loosely, it may be said that complementary therapies are used alongside conventional medicine, while alternative healthcare may be used instead of it. However, particularly with children, no professional practitioner would advise against giving your child any necessary drugs. But with the guidance of that practitioner, a child may be able to reduce or even eventually come off those drugs. For instance, in the case of eczema, many children who have been treated with one therapy, traditional Chinese medicine, have been able to stop using strong creams containing steroids.

Complementary therapies don't usually offer a 'quick cure' like some drugs. Although sometimes they can have a beneficial effect after just one treatment, they generally need to be used for at least three sessions to be able to get to work properly. As the whole wellbeing of the child is being looked at, the immune system will probably need building up and this takes time.

If after about three sessions though, you feel the therapy is doing nothing to help your child, then maybe you should try something different. Just as one drug may not work for a child, so some therapies work better on one individual than others.

Making the Decision

It can be difficult to decide to try something 'alternative' for your child. Although many parents are against having to give their child drugs, many feel they are not informed enough about complementary medicine to try it.

Before writing this book, I had talked to many parents – family friends, mothers met through antenatal classes, parents interviewed for magazine articles and so on, who were interested in complementary medicine, but felt they didn't know enough about it to entrust their child to an unknown practitioner.

There are many questions they wanted to ask before deciding to try a complementary therapy. Which one will suit their child best, where do they find someone who is not a quack, but a fully qualified practitioner, what will happen during an appointment, how much will it cost and is it available on the NHS? Hopefully this book can answer those questions. It can seem strange when first visiting an alternative or complementary practitioner. Instead of a GP's ten-minute consultation, the practitioner will spend around an hour asking questions, wanting to know everything there is to know about your child before making a diagnosis. They may seem unusual questions and, to you, totally irrelevant if you've taken your child for say, persistent ear ache, but the practitioner is building up a detailed picture.

Getting Referral on the NHS

You should always consult your GP first if you have any worries about your child's health. And if you do decide to try an alternative alongside conventional medicine, let your GP know. Local GPs are becoming more and more aware of the benefits of complementary therapies being used in conjunction or instead of their own treatment. For instance, a GP will know that a child's football injury could well be better treated by a chiropractor or osteopath than what he or she could offer.

A recent independent study carried out by the Medical Care Research Unit of the University of Sheffield on behalf of the Department of Health found that almost 40 per cent of GP partnerships in England provide access to one of the forms of complementary medicine (unfortunately the study did not cover the whole of the UK). And nearly a quarter of all GP referrals of those questioned were for a complementary therapy.

GPs can either refer you to an independent therapist, or some practices employ therapists on-site who are available at certain times during surgery hours. This is more likely if the GP is in a fund-holding practice. And increasingly, some GPs are also training as complementary therapists themselves. Although it may seem ideal to be able to see your GP for both conventional and complementary healthcare, always check how much training they have undergone. A few short courses in acupuncture do not compare to the years of training and clinical practice a fully qualified alternative practitioner has done.

But, on a wider scale, those in charge of the NHS health authorities are also cautiously looking at the 'unconventional'. A survey into complementary therapies in the NHS carried out by NAHAT (National Association of Health Authorities and Trusts) found that although many local health authorities had a positive attitude to complementary therapies, particularly the more recognized ones such as acupuncture, osteopathy, chiropractic and homoeopathy, they didn't really know a lot about them, there were reservations about their use within the NHS and there was an obvious reluctance to spend budgets on 'alternatives'.

Complementary therapies might seem alternative, but many of them, such as traditional Chinese medicine, acupuncture, reflexology and so on have been around for thousands of years, while others over a hundred years. If they hadn't proved successful for so many people they would have fallen out of use well before now.

Some parents have found a therapy has had a wonderful effect on their child, improving or curing a condition that has caused misery for months or years. Others have found they helped little. But when it comes to the health of your child, isn't it worth trying?

The Purpose of This Book

The aim of this book is to highlight the alternatives open to you when looking after the health of your child. It is intended as a guide to which therapies may be able to help a variety of common childhood complaints. The suggestions within each therapy listed in Section I: The Ailments are there as a guide to what a practitioner may prescribe and are not meant as advice on what to buy as a home remedy. Having said that, for some of the minor complaints (such as a sting), you would not need to go, for example, to an aromatherapist; the complaint could be easily treated at home. In these occasional instances, tips for home use have been included.

Notes

- The names of any remedies included under each ailment

such as homoeopathy, herbal medicine, Chinese medicine or aromatherapy etc. are listed as a guide to what a practitioner may give your child and are not meant as a guide to what to buy over the counter. You should always consult a qualified practitioner first who will decide on treatment only after careful analysis of your child.

- If you do buy any remedies over the counter, always follow any instructions and cautions carefully. There are also many good books on particular complementary therapies which can give you a more in-depth knowledge (see Section II: The Therapies). If you are in any doubt about your child's health, consult your practitioner or doctor.

- Under the traditional Chinese medicine entries, for ease of understanding, the common name rather than Chinese name has been used in most cases. If there is no common name the Chinese or botanical name has been used.

SECTION I

The Ailments

ABSCESSES, dental (gum boil)

This pus-filled sac develops when bacteria invade the soft tissue at the root of a decaying tooth. Symptoms can include throbbing pain, tender and inflamed gums and swelling, sometimes accompanied by headache and fever. This is distressing and uncomfortable for any child, and treatment, usually involving antibiotics, should be prompt to reduce the risk of loosing a tooth or septicaemia (blood poisoning) developing. Quick treatment is particularly important if it develops in a primary tooth, as it may damage the permanent tooth underneath. Once the boil has burst and the pus begins to seep away, the pain should lessen.

What you can do

If you believe your child is developing an abscess, consult your doctor or dentist. To help your child until then, rinse the mouth out with a weak solution of warm water and salt (although ensure that they are old enough not to swallow it, as salt solutions can cause kidney damage in young children). A gargle with a few drops of Tea-Tree oil added to water may also be beneficial. As a preventative measure in the future, a balanced diet is one of the best ways to promote healthy teeth and gums. Feed children plenty of fruit and vegetables and keep sweets and cakes to a minimum. Make teeth-cleaning a fun time rather than a chore – lead by example, even if it means brushing your own teeth more than usual. Children should be taken regularly to the dentist from the age of three.

Treatment

Medical attention should be sought, but the following complementary therapies may also be beneficial:

Herbal medicine A herbalist will be able to treat the abscess alongside any antibiotics recommended by your child's doctor or dentist. Immune-stimulating herbs such as Myrrh may be given. This may be given in tincture form, such as ten drops in a glass of water, to be rinsed in the mouth three times a day for as long as necessary.

Naturopathy A naturopath may see an abscess as a sign of toxicity in your child. This could be due to a diet too high in sugar and fats and the abscess is the body's way of releasing the toxins. The child's immune system will probably be low, so building this up with a balanced diet will be advised. Supplement mineral salts, such as potassium chloride, iron and calcium phosphate, may be suggested, depending on any other symptoms, combined with an increase of vitamin C. Foods that can puncture the gums such as crisps should be avoided. If antibiotics have been prescribed, live bio-yoghurt or the supplement acidophilus will be recommended to help boost healthy bacteria in the bowel.

Acupuncture Acupuncturists see abscesses and boils as an accumulation of what they term as damp phlegm and stagnation in the body and would treat the causes of these rather than the abscess itself. They may not treat a child with acupuncture with an abscess present as it can often be painful using localized points, but some may use distal points on the hand, which affect the mouth and gums, and is often used in dentistry. But they can also treat a child to help prevent future reoccurrence.

Caution

It's not advisable to lance the boil yourself to release the pus as this could lead to further infection. Consult your doctor or practitioner.

ACNE

Young teenagers can be afflicted by spots which can leave them feeling self-conscious and embarrassed. The spots, in the form of blackheads or whiteheads, are caused by an increase in the production of sebum brought on by the hormonal changes at puberty. Too much sebum can build up, blocking pores and resulting in pimples which can become infected, leading to bigger and more unsightly eruptions. But squeezing too often can lead to pitting and scars that can remain for life.

What you can do

Tempting though it may be, advise your child not to squeeze the spots, as this can lead to infection. Keep the skin as clean as possible by washing it three or four times a day, but without letting the skin dry out – a non-oily, water-based moisturizer will help. Cider vinegar – one dessertspoon (10ml) in a cup of hot water – drunk first thing in the morning and last thing at night, may help.

Treatment

Naturopathy A naturopath may recommend washing with an organic Dead Sea soap. Any excess facial oil still remaining can be gently removed by wiping the area with cotton wool soaked in witch hazel or a small amount of neat Tea-Tree oil. Although the main cause of acne is usually hormonal, stress, a low immune system and diet are also important. To help fight against infection, meals should contain raw or lightly cooked vegetables, grilled rather than fried foods, and plenty of wholegrains. Avoid animal fats, refined products and processed oils, except quality vegetable oils. There may be a link between acne and the chemicals added to salt found in fast and convenience foods. There is also some evidence that acne sufferers have a zinc deficiency, so an increase in zinc (found in chicken, fish, wholegrains, shellfish) or in supplement form may help. A well-balanced diet should provide all the vitamins needed to help the skin heal.

Traditional Chinese medicine A practitioner may see the

appearance of acne as the result of phlegm building up from unresolved problems earlier in childhood. At puberty, the Chinese see the Qi, or vital energy, and blood as being in a state of excess, which can affect the stomach, lungs and large intestines and erupt in the face. Your child will be encouraged to drink plenty of water as an eliminant, as well as looking carefully at the diet. Cooling herbs will be given to resolve this heat excess. Treatment may also include acupuncture, if necessary. Western herbal medicine might advise infusions of stinging nettle, burdock, dandelion, chamomile or onion, or lotions containing thyme, marigold or angelica. Eating a clove of garlic a day is also thought beneficial.

Kinesiology A kinesiologist would look for any imbalances in the body and for any mineral or vitamin deficiencies which can lead to skin problems. Advice on diet and lifestyle would hope to help rectify the problem.

Bach Flower Remedies Two drops of Crab Apple diluted in an egg-cup full of water and dabbed on the affected area with cotton wool morning and evening has helped some sufferers. If the acne is causing a lack of self confidence, Larch should help, while Gorse will help restore a feeling of optimism to those who are convinced that nothing can be done to help them.

Other therapies that may be beneficial: aromatherapy, herbal medicine, homoeopathy, reflexology, biochemic tissue salts.

'I'd read about applied kinesiology in a magazine article. Janice was suffering terribly with acne – it was particularly bad on her forehead and was making her really introverted because she was so embarrassed, even though we told her most kids go through it. She tried every cream sold in the chemist and the doctor had even put her on a course of antibiotics to get rid of them, but nothing seemed to work for her. So we thought we'd give it a go and I said I'd pay for her to try the kinesiology. She had several treatments which worked on balancing the bowel. They found she also had a zinc deficiency and once these two were rectified, her skin started getting better. I was told that coffee was aggravating her skin – she'd always loved it from a young age – and that she was dehydrated. So she cut down on the coffee and drank more water. It took a few months, but her skin completely cleared up. For the first time in her life she could wear her hair without a fringe!'

Terri and Janice, now 14

AGGRESSION

There can be many reasons for aggressiveness in a child. It may just be their nature or a phase they are going through where they feel perhaps they are not getting enough attention and want their voices heard. However, there may be a particular reason for a sudden change of character. Aggression at home towards siblings may be a child's way of retaliating against being bullied at school. They may be bored or understimulated and need an outlet for their energy. Or, possibly an allergy to a particular food or medicine may be causing irritability.

What you can do

Try to find out if there is a reason behind any aggression – whether it can be linked to any recent event, such as starting school or eating certain foods. If it seems it may just be a passing problem, your child will hopefully be able to work things out for themselves. But more deepseated problems may need further help.

Treatment

Hypnotherapy Methods of hypnotherapy vary, but the

hypnotherapist may use a series of techniques which will help the child to learn about their behaviour without being aware of actually doing so. The hypnotherapist will concentrate on the positive aspects and try to break associations with negative aspects in the child's life. They will then be taught how to use those positive times in their present life.

Osteopathy A difficult birth or an accident can all play a part in the development of a child. If the cerebral areas responsible for the child's personality and communication are affected, then this can lead to problems such as aggression. An osteopath will work on these areas to release any suppression. Often the pathways responsible for behaviour are disfunctioning and need awakening and reinforcing to help the child.

Bach Flower Remedies A strong-willed child who likes to get their own way on their own terms may benefit from Vine. Where the aggression is based on hatred, spite or jealousy, Holly may be given, while children who fly into uncontrolled rages would benefit from Cherry Plum.

Other therapies that may be beneficial: massage, reflexology, traditional Chinese medicine, naturopathy.

ALLERGIES

Allergies occur when the body has an abnormal reaction to a substance or *allergen*. Allergies are caused by any number of things – foods (such as dairy products, shellfish and nuts), animal fur, dust, pollen or chemicals – and is the body's way of fighting off what it thinks are foreign invaders. Allergies can cause asthma, eczema, hayfever, rashes (see under relevant alphabetical section) or, on rare occasions, anaphylactic shock (see Caution) after being stung by an insect or after having eaten a particular food, such as peanuts.

When the body thinks it is being attacked by foreign invaders, it reacts by releasing antibodies. As the allergens and antibodies fight it out, this causes the release of chemicals, including histamine, which will result in the allergic symptoms. Depending on what has been eaten/inhaled/touched, this can result in an itchy rash and dry skin as in eczema; narrowing of the airways and difficulty in breathing, as in asthma; sneezing and runny nose, as in hayfever; or vomiting and diarrhoea as in food allergy. Other symptoms can include headache, wheezing, catarrh and watery eyes.

For an allergy to occur, your child will already have to have come into contact with the allergen once before. So, for instance, the first time your child stroked a cat would not have caused problems, but the second time could trigger an allergy.

Allergies tend to run in families, so if you or your partner suffer, your child is more susceptible.

What you can do

Unfortunately, cases of allergies, particularly asthma and hayfever, are on the increase. With rising pollution levels from industry and car exhaust fumes, there's not always a lot you can do to avoid them, but you can minimize exposure to some.

- Breastfeed for as long as possible to help your child build up immunity.
- If you know your child is allergic to a certain food, cut out the offending food from their diet and check all food labels. Let their school and other parents know.
- Keep bedrooms clean, regularly vacuuming the mattress and all soft furnishings, including curtains, where dust mites – a common allergen – live. It also helps to use synthetic (non-feather) duvets and pillows and to cover

mattresses, pillows and duvets with dust proof covers. Wash all bedding weekly in a hot wash (60° C).

- Contact with cleaning products (although these should be kept locked up anyway) can cause reactions. Thoroughly rinse the bath or sink after cleaning.
- If your child seems to break out in a rash after a hug from you, it could be a reaction to your perfume or deodorant.
- Ionizers release negative ions into the atmosphere to counter positive ions which can lead to headaches and irritability, and may be useful for asthmatics. They cost from about £35 from chemists, electrical or natural health stores.

Treatment

Kinesiology This therapy is most well known for identifying allergies. It is said to take the guess-work out of finding which foods your child is sensitive to. Muscle testing is used to assess the body's response to each food that is introduced by placing a small amount between the lips or holding it in the hand. The muscle will either stay strong or weaken if the food is having a detrimental effect. Kinesiologists see food sensitivities as a symptom, not a cause, of illness. When a child is stressed or unwell, they are more likely to develop a reaction to a food, usually one they eat most of, such as wheat or dairy products. Kinesiologists may suggest excluding the offending food and will also work on building up the immune and endocrine systems with treatment and nutrition. Once the symptoms are relieved, the body will get back to optimum health over a few months and then the food may be retested and reintroduced to the diet if there are no problems.

Homoeopathy A homoeopath may prescribe Sulphur for an itchy rash, Euphrasia for itchy, watering eyes or Nat. mur. for a runny nose, to suit your child. A change of diet and lifestyle may also be recommended, depending on the type of allergy. In case of severe food allergy, as e.g. with nuts, which can cause anaphylactic shock and even be fatal, Apis mel. can be beneficial.

Herbal medicine A herbalist may recommend an infusion of Elderflower, which has decongestant properties which can help to loosen phlegm and also acts as a relaxant to calm the nerves and allay any anxieties the child may be feeling about their allergy. Other herbs such as Eyebright which works as an anti-inflammatory and astringent and Plantain which has useful expectorant properties may also be advised.

Acupuncture One study found that giving patients acupuncture before the pollen season started was successful in nearly 70 per cent of cases and in some cases the success achieved lasted for more than three years. Although acupuncturists understand the use of allergy testing so that allergens can be identified and avoided, they will want to find the underlying reason or cause for the allergy surfacing in the first place, such as what they see as a deficiency of energy in the spleen or kidney. This may be due to not sleeping, a lack of fresh fruit and vegetables or they may see it as acquiring too much static electricity from being too close to a TV set for too long.

Caution

An extreme allergic reaction, known as anaphylactic shock, when the victim suffers a sudden lowering of blood pressure, may cause them to pass out. Other symptoms include difficulty in breathing, due to airways narrowing, swelling of the tongue or throat, pain in the abdomen and diarrhoea. Immediate medical attention should be sought.

Other therapies that may be beneficial: traditional Chinese medicine, yoga, Bach Flower Remedies, osteopathy.

'Sam is our only child and was a really happy, easy-going little boy. But a few months ago he started being disruptive at school and began to sleep badly, coughing all night. Then he got a rash all over his torso, which I was afraid was eczema. I took him to an acupuncturist who told me that he had a deficient kidney yin which was causing what the Chinese call empty heat.

'The acupuncturist asked a lot of questions about Sam – his health, his likes and dislikes, our family background. I had to admit that my husband and I were having serious problems in our marriage. The acupuncturist felt that the tension at home was having an effect on Sam. It explained his behaviour at school and the rash was a physical sign of his being upset. The fact he kept waking up in the night was also a subconscious attempt to stay awake and be with us as inside he was afraid. The acupuncturist said night time is yin time and if he spent a lot of time awake he was becoming more yin deficient. Usually his body would have fought off any triggers to a rash, but because of the deficiency, he couldn't cope. He was treated for the rash and then to build up the deficiency so that he's better able to cope with the difficulties we're having at home.'

Alison and Sam, 6

ANXIETY

Children can experience anxiety from a very young age. Whether it's first being parted from their mother, starting a new school, being bullied or suffering the effects of parental divorce. Anxiety can manifest itself in a number of physical problems including bedwetting, headaches, nightmares, disruptive behaviour and skin problems. Although these can all be treated (see under relevant alphabetical section) the root cause of the anxiety also needs to be looked at and treated.

What you can do
Try to ensure that your child feels they have a secure, stable home and loving parents, even – or particularly – when there may be marital discord. If your child suddenly develops unexplained ailments, set aside time to sit and talk on a one-to-one basis to find any possible root to a problem that might seem totally unrelated.

Treatment
Bach Flower Remedies These work well as the Remedies are chosen as a result of the child's emotional and mental health rather than for a specific problem. For an acute anxiety attack, the general Rescue Remedy is helpful. If the child is anxious about something specific, such as travelling or a test at school, Mimulus may help. If the child lacks confidence and worries about failing, Larch may be beneficial and Aspen may be given if the child has vague fears and forebodings that do not seem to have any definite cause.

Aromatherapy Aromatherapy oils have wonderful therapeutic qualities. Two or three drops of Sandalwood, Ylang-ylang, Lavender or Geranium in the bath or on your child's pillow may help to soothe (beware over-use of Ylang-ylang as this can be a stimulant). Massaging your child with oils will not only relax them but it will allow them time to forget any worries or let them out in the open, if they feel like talking. One study found that children suffering from anxiety and depression had reduced symptoms after being massaged for half an hour each day, and that they slept for longer periods each night.

Kinesiology Kinesiologists believe that anxiety might not just lie in the mind. It may be a physical problem that manifests as anxiety. It may be something the child is eating that is causing the problem, or an emotional problem, leading to their energy levels becoming blocked. Applying kinesiology will help to find the body's imbalances and working on one imbalance may be the key to detecting and treating others.

Hypnotherapy The hypnotherapist will help the child to look at the times when they become anxious, for instance going to school, and to try and cut the connection between those times and the negative feelings of anxiety, while at the same time suggesting positive emotions.

Other therapies that may be beneficial: osteopathy, acupressure, massage, herbal medicine, homoeopathy, yoga.

'My son Richard always leaves his homework to the last minute and then gets completely worked up when he realizes how much he has to do in how little time. Recently, he spent all weekend saying he had no work to do until Sunday night when he admitted he had maths, art and English to get through. He didn't know where to start and became more and more anxious about getting it all done. I sat him down at the table with his books and brought him a glass of orange juice with a couple of drops of Elm flower remedy, which works well for the feeling of being overwhelmed. The doorbell went and when I returned to him five minutes later, it was a different boy sitting there. He'd rationalized what he needed to do, sorted out all his books, decided what had to be worked on first and what could wait and was getting on with it. Children respond really well to Bach Flower Remedies – they're like sponges, taking all they need from them.'

Alison and Richard, 12

ASTHMA

Asthma is a common disease, and its occurrence is growing due to factors such as increasingly poor air quality and growing incidence of food intolerance thought to be related to the use of pesticides and drugs. About one in seven children suffer. It is commonly caused by allergens such as pollen, housedust, animals or feathers. An allergic reaction to these allergens causes breathlessness and wheezing as the bronchioles – the small airways in the lung – narrow. Mucus secretion also increases, which further blocks the airways. Exercise, emotional upset, smoke or an infection can also cause an attack. Your child is also more likely to suffer if asthma or a related allergy such as eczema or hayfever runs in the family.

Some asthma attacks may be mild while others are severe. During an attack, children can become very distressed as they fight for breath, making the problem worse. They may cough to try and remove the mucus and may go blue around the lips due to lack of oxygen. Some children have persistent coughing, particularly during the night, especially young children.

What you can do

Identify which allergens are causing problems. In the bedroom, regularly clean the mattress, soft furnishings and curtains and hot wash linens to minimize dust mites. Keep the windows at home and in the car closed during high pollen counts. Eliminate any foods that may be at fault, although this should only be done under supervision. Try to minimize stressful situations, if these are a trigger. And, sad though it may be, if you have pets try to see whether contact with them brings on an attack. Swimming is known to be a good exercise that can strengthen the lungs without too much overexertion.

During an attack, sit your child up, propped up by (nonfeather) pillows and try to keep them as calm as possible. If you're looking anxious yourself this will only transmit to the child. (See also Allergies and Hayfever.)

Treatment

Medical attention should be sought, but the following complementary therapies may also be beneficial:

Traditional Chinese medicine TCM has proved successful for many asthmatics, with some finding that acupuncture or acupressure have helped reduce attacks. There have been many studies carried out on childhood asthma where acupuncture has, in some cases, significantly improved symptoms. Herbs may also be prescribed to help resolve what TCM sees as weakness in the lung, spleen or kidney and too much phlegm. Other herbs may be given for use during an attack, once the child's 'pattern' of attacks is understood. Other herbs will be given to protect from colds and allergic attacks, such as ginseng, liquorice, angelica and apricot. A diet including plenty of fresh fruit and vegetables, oily fish, garlic and onions and steering clear of refined foods, dairy products and additives and colourings, such as tartrazine, may all help to reduce symptoms.

Naturopathy This may include a number of therapies. A naturopath may advise a diet that includes fresh vegetables and fruit (but avoiding citrus), wholemeal foods and cutting back or preferably cutting out dairy and refined products. Garlic and onions may be recommended as they are said to help counter the production of mucus, and reducing eating red meat to once or twice a week may be advised. Osteopathy or gentle massage, to help loosen the chest muscles and joints to ease breathing, and a gentle exercise programme to increase respiratory strength may also be advised. Your child will also be assessed for food allergies, for instance to dairy products, wheat or foods containing additives. Mineral salt supplements, such as calcium and magnesium phosphate, may be recommended, to help support the body.

Homoeopathy One recent study found homoeopathy very successful in treating bronchial asthma. A combination of remedies may be used, but a homoeopath will treat each child as an individual, depending on their particular condition. So, Phosphorus may be given to deal with wheezing and coughing. If your child is affected by dust and the drying effects of central heating and suffers wheezing and shortness of breath, which is worse at night, Kali. Carb. may be prescribed and so on.

Chiropractic A chiropractor may be able to help with strain and stiffness caused by heavy and difficult breathing. They will correct any stiffness in the joints and muscles of the midback and ribcage. This will not only help with the physical effort of breathing but can help stimulate the nervous supply to those joints, muscles and also the lungs.

Osteopathy An osteopath may be able to improve the workings of the chest and the functions of the spine, ribs and diaphragm through manipulation. Cranial work may also be done to rebalance any interference in the body's system which controls involuntary actions which may lead to excess mucus secretion, causing congestion and constricted lung tissue.

Caution

During an attack or when symptoms are severe, always consult a doctor. You should always have the prescribed orthodox drugs at home, ready to administer. Once you have discussed your child's health with a complementary practitioner, you can decide together how to move forward in treating your child's illness.

Other therapies that may be beneficial: yoga, hypnotherapy, herbal medicine, Alexander Technique, Bach Flower Remedies.

'When Oona was about fourteen months old we woke up one night to hear her gasping for breath. We rushed her to hospital where she was treated and it was explained that she probably had asthma. When it happened again we were told that she'd have to be put permanently on medication and that she'd have to have steroids to prevent further attacks.

'We decided to try homoeopathy as we didn't like the thought that she'd have to take drugs for the rest of her life. I really didn't know anything about homoeopathy, but a friend's child had successfully been treated for eczema with it, so we thought we'd give it a go. On the first visit we spent two hours talking about Oona's health – everything from her birth to which antibiotics she'd had. Can you imagine a doctor having time to do that, even if you did go privately! We were just asked to pay whatever we could afford to.

'We were warned that the remedy would first bring out the symptoms and that Oona would get worse before she got better. Even so it was quite traumatic. But there were longer spaces between each attack. I called the homoeopath every day and she was really supportive. In the end though, we did stop the homoeopathy, and occasionally she goes back on the medication. I just felt I wanted to wait until Oona was older and more resilient to attacks.'

Louise and Oona, 2½

ATHLETE'S FOOT

This fungal infection thrives in moist conditions and is usually found between the toes, making them dry and itchy, and also sometimes affects the nails. The affected skin may eventually peel off. It is more common in older children and the infection can be picked up in damp areas such as changing rooms or swimming pools. It develops when the feet become sweaty and don't have a chance to breathe and dry out.

What you can do

Let children go barefoot or wear sandals when they can to allow air to circulate around the feet. Cotton socks are preferable to cotton mix or synthetics. After bathing, always dry feet thoroughly, particularly between the toes. If the infection is already present, keep floors clean and don't let children share towels to reduce the risk of passing on infection.

Treatment

Traditional Chinese medicine A practitioner may give a mixture of herbs to treat the condition and build up the immune system to combat further infection. They may also advise immersing the foot in a bowl of hot water with 575ml vinegar and two crushed garlic cloves, used for their antifungal properties, for about twenty to thirty minutes, which should be repeated until the condition clears up.

Herbal medicine Golden seal root is known for its antibacterial and viral properties and may be recommended by a herbalist. A suggestion may be to add half a teaspoon of golden seal to a cup of boiling water and let it stand for 5–10 minutes. Then add the mixture to a bowl of tepid water and soak the affected foot for 5 minutes. Or Calendula in cream form, which has antifungal properties, may help.

Aromatherapy There are a number of essential oils which may be given to help treat athlete's foot. Tea-Tree oil works well on any fungal infection and also has antiseptic properties. Lavender can help to regenerate new skin growth and Geranium has cleansing properties and works well for most skin conditions.

Other therapies that may be beneficial: naturopathy, acupuncture, homoeopathy.

ATTENTION DEFICIT DISORDER (ADD)

This disorder, although not new, has been the subject of much recent debate. ADD is another term for hyperactivity, and although many parents might loosely claim their child is hyperactive, ADD is thought to be hereditary and is caused by a minor disorder of the brain, which fails to stop unreasonable behaviour. It mildly affects about 10 per cent of children and 2 per cent more severely. More boys than girls are affected and problems are more noticeable once the child has started school. Symptoms can include inattention, overactivity, impulsiveness which leads to accidents, insatiability and social ineptitude. It affects the child's learning and behavioural abilities, causing problems in lessons and in the playground. This in itself can cause problems as the child feels stupid and left out by his classmates. Over half the children affected also have specific learning difficulties such as dyslexia.

What you can do

Many parents feel they are inadequate to deal with such a disruptive child and that they are in some way to blame. But there are ways of making life easier. Accept your child as they are – and accept that they are different. Provide routines and guidelines so they know where they stand and let them know what you want in calm and simple language. Try to avoid possible triggers of outbursts such as long car journeys, keeping situations as stress-free as possible. Emphasize and reward the good in them rather than concentrating on the bad. And if things do get out of control, have a room or a chair for 'time out' where they are sent until they've quietened down.

Treatment

Naturopathy Although it is generally agreed that diet does have some part to play in ADD, there are differing opinions as to how large a part that is. But some studies have shown that food intolerance can be a cause of hyperkinetic activity in children. Additives, natural and manufactured preservatives, chocolate, strawberries, cola, colourings and flavourings may all cause problems. A naturopath may advise an exclusion diet, to be carried out under supervision, where the numbers of foods eaten are restricted and then slowly reintroduced.

Hypnotherapy Therapists use a variety of techniques to treat attention deficit disorder, depending on their particular training. They may use a series of approaches so that the child unconsciously learns how they should be behaving. Just as it is a natural process for children to learn to talk, it can be a natural process for them to learn again how to behave.

Osteopathy An osteopath may carry out certain structural mechanical treatments and massage to help calm down the child. Cranial osteopathic techniques may be able to help problems caused by foetal development, a difficult birth or an accident which can affect functioning. Cerebral areas which are associated with or responsible for the child's personality or communication skills may have been suppressed. The central nervous system and cranial system which control movement may also have been affected and will be looked at.

Traditional Chinese medicine Studies have shown the effectiveness of treating hyperactivity with TCM. Some have shown great improvement in behaviour, attention span and academic records; some even being completely cured. A TCM practitioner will need to know exactly how the child acts before deciding on treatment.

'Keith became very difficult when his father left home, and his behaviour got worse when my present partner moved in. You couldn't hold his attention for more than two minutes, then he'd be off, doing something else or just deliberately not listening.

'He became very disruptive at school, annoying the other kids, shouting in class, talking back to the teachers. He had no friends he was so unsociable. I could just feel all the parents and teachers thinking "why can't she control her son?"

'He was sent to an educational psychologist once a week for two years, but it didn't do a thing to help. A teacher suggested that he try hypnotherapy. By this time I was sceptical that anything could help, but I agreed to let him try it.

'Through five sessions he began to focus on the positive things that had happened in his life rather than the negative. He became a lot more relaxed, he was able to concentrate on things – start a project and actually finish it off. He had been way behind in his schoolwork, but within about six months his reading skills had caught up by two years.

'He's such a relaxed, happy child now. He has friends round all the time – I can't get rid of them. I just look at him and think, where did this easy-going, co-operative child come from? He's wonderful.'

Barbara and Keith, 12

BACK PAIN

There can be many causes of back pain or backache. Part, or all of the back may hurt and if muscles have been affected, the surrounding tissue may also become inflamed, causing further pain. Your child may have just moved awkwardly, pulling a muscle or straining a joint. Lifting heavy objects, sports, over-exertion or illness such as 'flu can all cause aches and pains which may just last a day or for much longer. It might also be the sign of a more serious problem, such as part of the spine being compressed, or the nerve roots affected.

What you can do
Get your child to rest as much as possible. If the pain seems

more than just a pulling of a joint or overstretching a muscle, consult your doctor for underlying causes.

Treatment

Chiropractic There can be many possible causes for upper, mid and lower back pain. A chiropractor will, as far as possible, eliminate any serious causes before starting treatment. If a structural cause is found, the chiropractor will correct the joints and muscles that are not functioning properly, with techniques appropriate to the child's age and the areas concerned. These may include spinal manipulation, mobilization, soft tissue therapy, exercise and ergonomic advice.

Kinesiology Kinesiologists believe that one of the sure ways of preventing backpain is to drink plenty of water. It is thought that drinking at least six glasses of water a day can help to hydrate the muscles and can sometimes completely relieve pain. The abdominal muscles will also be looked at as they can be affected by lower backache. Neuro-lymphatic massage may be used to balance the muscles and therefore strengthen the back.

Osteopathy An osteopath will look for any causes behind backache, such as problems with posture or the mechanics of the spine. This may be due to a local problem as a result of a fall, for instance, or due to overstraining the spine because of a problem elsewhere in the body. The osteopath will gently correct any misalignments of the spine, pelvis and limbs, allowing the body to heal and alleviating symptoms.

Other therapies that may be beneficial: Alexander Technique, yoga, reflexology, massage, acupuncture.

BEDWETTING

This is an upsetting problem for children, particularly older ones, but there are treatments that have worked successfully.

By three or four years old, 85 per cent of children are dry through the night, except for the occasional accident. At the age of five, around 10 per cent will still be wetting the bed. By age fifteen, only a few – about 2 per cent – will still bed-wet. The cause may be lack of bladder control or it can be related to stress and anxiety. A six-year-old who may have been dry throughout the night may suddenly start again after the arrival of a new baby in the household. An older child may have problems at school which are causing unconscious distress.

What you can do

Whatever the reason for bedwetting, time, patience and understanding are needed rather than admonishment. Don't make an issue of it with young children when changing the sheets. Older children may prefer to do this themselves to save embarrassment. Using waterproof sheets will help protect the mattress.

Buzzers have proved successful in many cases. At the start of urinating, the buzzer goes off, waking the child, who can then go to the loo.

Treatment

Chiropractic A chiropractor would first check for congenital and hereditary problems before treatment. They may then work on the lower back and pelvis to stimulate the nervous supply to the urinary system, which may help to alleviate symptoms. One study found that chiropractic helped 25 per cent of those treated for bedwetting by 50 per cent or more.

Osteopathy An osteopath may check for irritation of the bladder or interference with its nerve supply which can be caused by bone misalignment. By correcting any relevant spinal and pelvic bone misalignment, the bedwetting may be cured.

Hypnotherapy Studies have found hypnotherapy effective in the treatment of bedwetting. One survey of boys aged eight–thirteen years old found six weekly sessions were significantly effective in reducing symptoms. Different approaches may be used, depending on the training of the therapist. Bedwetting often begins at a time of stress, for instance parents' marital break-up. But rather than getting the child to remember this difficult time and remembering the cause, they will try to help the child disassociate bedtime with wetting the bed, so that the child can see night time as a time for sleeping rather than wetting.

Traditional Chinese medicine A Chinese doctor may identify bedwetting as the disruption of fluid circulating in the kidney, spleen and lungs. Herbs which act as toners and astringents may be given, but the doctor will also try to identify the possible underlying cause of insecurity in the child. There have been many positive studies into the use of acupuncture (also used in Chinese medicine) and bedwetting. One survey showed that seven out of ten children treated were cured of the problem after a course of acupuncture and a further two had improved conditions.

Caution

If there seems to be no underlying causes for the incontinence consult a doctor, as a bladder infection or abnormality might be the problem.

Other therapies that may be beneficial: Bach Flower Remedies, homoeopathy.

BITES/STINGS (insects)

Insect bites and stings are rarely a real problem unless they become infected, your child has an allergic reaction or they occur abroad where a disease such as malaria is present. However, they can be very sore and itchy, and in the case of an allergic reaction, cause the area to swell up.

What you can do

If still embedded, carefully remove the sting. Don't use tweezers as this will squeeze the sting, releasing more venom.

If you know your child is allergic to bee, wasp or hornet stings, antihistamine or alternative remedies should be available at all times during the summer. Immediate action is also needed if the child is stung in the mouth or throat, as these may swell and hinder breathing. If this happens, and the child is old enough, give them ice cubes to suck and get medical help.

Treatment

Aromatherapy Eucalyptus oil – about four or five drops diluted in a cup of water and dabbed on exposed areas – acts as a natural insect repellent. The antiseptic qualities of Tea-Tree oil gently rubbed on to the sting will help soothe it.

Traditional Chinese medicine TCM and Western methods of treatment are often similar. A practitioner may administer crushed Marigold leaves to reduce the effect of the sting. TCM believes wasp stings are alkaline, so can be neutralized by a mild acid, such as lemon juice or vinegar. Bee stings are acidic, so an alkaline remedy such as bicarbonate of soda, may be effective. Tea-Tree and Lavender can also help to soothe.

Homoeopathy A homoeopath may recommend Apis for pain and swelling, Cantharis, for the hot, burning sensation and Ledum if the child is feeling particularly sensitive and to prevent infection.

Herbal medicine A herbalist may recommend a variety of remedies to help soothe the bite or sting. An Aloe Vera gel, which has cooling properties, may help. Or a dab of Lavender oil applied to the area will help the healing process. Chamomile cream will help to soothe.

Caution

For severe allergic reactions, resulting in anaphylactic shock where breathing becomes difficult, the throat swells and the child may collapse, immediate medical attention is needed and a shot of adrenaline may be given. Emergency self-injection kits are available for those known to be at risk.

BLISTERS

Although not usually a serious problem, blisters can be uncomfortable for active children and so the quicker they clear up, the better. Blisters are made up of fluid that collects beneath the skin, forming a raised area. The fluid forms after minor damage to the area, such as friction from a rubbing shoe or a burn.

What you can do

Blisters are best left to heal alone, as the sterile fluid acts as protection and pricking can leave them open to infection. If pricking it is necessary, use a sterilized needle (put the needle in a flame for a few seconds and then cool), drain the fluid and cover with a sterile dressing, although allow to air as much as possible.

Treatment

Traditional Chinese medicine A practitioner may recommend an infusion of Rosemary or Sage leaves applied to the area which will act as a soothing antiseptic.

Aromatherapy Chamomile Roman may be used for its antiseptic qualities, while Lavender soothes. A solution of two drops to half a cup of water, dabbed on to the blister should help.

Biochemic tissue salts Nat. mur. may be advised which can help to bring pain relief.

BRONCHIOLITIS

This acute infection, which can be serious, occurs when the bronchioles (the smallest airways in the lungs) become infected with a virus. It usually occurs in babies and is particularly dangerous in babies who have underlying lung or heart problems. It starts as a cold and then develops into fast and noisy breathing, accompanied by coughing. They may seem to be fighting for air and begin to go blue around the mouth. Fever and drowsiness may also be symptoms. There are epidemics during the winter every couple or so years. Hospital treatment is not always necessary, but if it is moderate to severe bronchiolitis then hospital admission may be advised as the baby may need oxygen as well as help with feeding. Sometimes artificial ventilation is necessary until breathing returns to normal. Bronchiolitis should clear up within a couple of weeks.

What you can do

If you see your baby is having difficulty in breathing, is looking blue around the mouth and has a temperature, consult a doctor immediately or take the baby to hospital for diagnosis.

Treatment

Medical attention should be sought, but the following complementary therapies may also be beneficial:

Homoeopathy Medical help should be sought immediately for bronchiolitis, but until help arrives or you take your child to hospital, try the following: if the child is wheezy, has a blue tinge and sounds hoarse, use Carbo. veg. 30c every ten minutes for up to ten doses. If the child is very weak from the effort of breathing, use Ant. tart. 30c.

Osteopathy To help aid recovery after bronchiolitis, an osteopath would hope to help improve the workings of the diaphragm, ribs and spine in the chest area and to work on the cranial area to clear any interference in the system that controls involuntary action such as the secretion of mucus. Advice may also be given on breathing, exercises and posture.

Traditional Chinese medicine Chinese medicine sees bronchiolitis as lung heat and phlegm heat and treatment will try to rebalance these. A range of herbs will be given during the early acute stages and others for the chronic stage, as it is important to clear the phlegm and help to stop the coughing. If the child suffers from repeated lung infections, they may be given jade screen powder from the end of summer to help prevent attacks through the winter.

BRONCHITIS

Bronchitis is inflammation of the larger airways or bronchi in the lungs. It may be caused by a cough or cold which causes the airways to become inflamed and swell, filling with phlegm. Although usually a viral condition, in which case treatment is not needed, it may be a bacterial infection. Your child may be taking rapid breaths which sound wheezy, have a dry cough, which as the chest becomes more congested, produces yellow or green phlegm, and may cause vomiting. They may feel worse at night. Other symptoms may include headache, loss of appetite, raised temperature and the lips and tongue may turn blueish.

What you can do
Encourage your child to cough up and spit out phlegm. Keep an eye on their temperature and sponge them down with tepid water (not cold) if it is high. Keep them quiet and warm and give them plenty of fluids to prevent dehydration. Putting your child across your lap, face down and patting them on the back may help during an attack of coughing.

Treatment
Homoeopathy The earlier the homoeopath can see your child, the quicker the treatment can start. At the first stage they may recommend Aconite, if the child has been exposed to cold, dry weather and biting wind. Bryonia will help with the dry,

painful cough after onset and if the child feels worse for movement. If the child has a hot, flushed face and dry hot skin and finds coughing is worse at night, Belladonna may be advised. When the phlegm is loosening up, but not being brought up by coughing, Ant. tart. may be used.

Acupuncture An acupuncturist may look for signs of 'cold' or 'hot' bronchitis. Cold bronchitis signs will be a child who is maybe already weak and the cold has gone to the lungs, which are not strong enough to expectorate the white-looking phlegm, while hot signs will be green or yellowy-green phlegm. If the phlegm is not properly cleared, it can recur weeks later. An acupuncturist will use various acupuncture points to clear the phlegm and strengthen the child so that in the future their body will be able to deal with it.

Reflexology A reflexologist may gently massage the foot before really going to work on it. The whole foot would be treated as the whole body will need to be brought back into balance to help the immune system fight infection. Particular attention would be paid to the throat, sinuses, eyes, ears and the lungs, as well as the solar plexus to include the diaphragm, small intestine, colon, spleen and spine to relax the chest muscles.

Caution

If you notice a blueish tinge around the lips or mouth, or if breathing is becoming more difficult, take them immediately to the doctor or hospital, as oxygen treatment may be needed.

Other therapies that may be beneficial: aromatherapy, naturopathy, osteopathy.

'I've been taking Amit to see an acupuncturist for the last year and a half. He's my last child and I had him late in life – when I was forty. He's always been weak and if he gets a cold it goes straight to his chest and he gets bronchitis. As much as his body is weak, his will is strong, and if he doesn't get his own way, tantrums always follow and he's rushing round everywhere screaming and shouting. It takes half an hour just to make him get into bed. He also likes to drink milk straight from the fridge. The acupuncturist uses all this information to build up an overall picture of his character and how to treat him.

'But it's taking a long while, even though he's a lot better. But every time we clear the phlegm, it returns the next time he's ill. He's being treated for the phlegm, but also to try and build up his strength so he can resist an infection next time.'

Nishma and Amit, now 5½

BRUISES

A bruise is usually due to a knock or fall. This causes a discolouration of the skin and sometimes a slight bump, as small blood vessels below the skin's surface temporarily leak blood. The bruise may first appear black or purple, but after a few days will turn yellow or green as the blood breaks down and the skin returns to normal.

What you can do
Most bruises need little or no treatment, but putting a cold compress over it for at least ten minutes should help to reduce the pain and swelling. If the skin is unbroken, Witch Hazel is also helpful.

Treatment
Aromatherapy Geranium, Rosemary, Lavender, Cypress and Eucalyptus all have qualities that can help contain the bruise. They can be applied in the form of a hot or cold compress, in combination totalling not more than six drops.
Homoeopathy A cream or lotion containing Arnica will help reduce bruising.

Bach Flower Remedies Rescue Remedy will help with the shock or trauma the child may be feeling after hurting themselves.

Caution

If pain caused by the bruise gets worse after twenty-four hours, or if it has not begun to fade after a few days, consult your doctor. It may be a sign of an underlying problem, such as a broken bone. If bruises appear on your child's body for no apparent reason, consult your doctor as this may be a sign of a more serious illness, such as haemophilia or leukaemia. *Other therapies that may be beneficial: acupuncture.*

BURNS/SCALDS (minor)

Many small burns or scalds are caused by intense heat, such as touching a hot pan, fire, hot liquid, electric current or staying too long in the sun (see under *Sunburn*). A minor burn will affect only the outer layer of the skin, causing it to redden and possibly blister. The damaged skin may peel off in a day or two. Only if you are sure that the burn or scald is minor should you treat it at home. If in any doubt, consult your doctor.

What you can do

Put the burn under cold running water, or gently apply a cold compress such as a soaked clean tea towel, for ten to fifteen minutes. Remove any restricting clothing or jewellery, being careful of the affected area. Cover the burns with a sterile dressing to keep it clean. Don't use adhesive plasters or apply butter as these may only make the condition worse and don't try to puncture the blister as this contains protective plasma. Give a pain-relieving remedy.

Treatment

Homoeopathy A number of remedies may be recommended

by a homoeopath, such as Cantharis, which works well for relieving pain and blistering, while Aconite will help the shock. If the burn begins to weep afterwards, Hep. sulph. may help, while Urtica Urens can also help minor burns which have blistered.

Bach Flower Remedies For the immediate shock, give Rescue Remedy or Star of Bethlehem. These can be taken by adding two drops of either to a glass of water, to be sipped throughout the day, or added to the water used in a cold compress.

Aromatherapy Mix a couple of drops of Lavender with Aloe Vera gel and apply to cool and soothe the area.

Herbal medicine A herbalist may recommend immediately applying Aloe Vera gel to cool and soothe the area. Then directly applying chopped-up Calendula flowers held in place with gauze may help. Calendula has antiseptic properties and can help the body to fight against infection. Elderflower, given in tea, will also help to relax and calm the child if they have been frightened by the burn as well as soothing the area.

Caution

A large proportion of the 1000 or so people admitted to hospital each year with burns or scalds are children who have had accidents in the home. More serious burns may be caused by touching, inhaling or drinking a chemical such as bleach or touching an electric current and will need *immediate* medical treatment, as deeper injuries can cause loss of body fluids from the affected area leading to lowered blood pressure, rapid pulse and shock. Emergency intravenous fluids may be necessary and drugs to prevent the infection.

'Emily usually knows not to touch the iron, but this time I think curiosity got the better of her. I'd been ironing shirts and some of the kids' clothes when the telephone went in the next room. I left the iron standing up on the board and went to answer it. Emily must have clambered on to the stool and was playing around, when she put her hand right across the hot plate.

'I heard this scream of anguish, dropped the phone and came running. I rushed her to the sink and kept her hand under cold running water for about ten minutes to take the heat out of the burn, while trying to calm her down. Then I put a drop of neat Lavender oil on to the area and repeated it an hour later. It wasn't actually as bad as I first thought, I think it just shocked Emily more than anything else. But the Lavender worked wonders – it's got antiseptic properties and can also act to kill pain. I know that it also helps the skin to regenerate, so it's particularly good for minor burns. No blister appeared and Emily didn't scar at all.' •

Beverley and Emily, 8

CHICKENPOX

Chickenpox is a common and generally mild infection caused by the varicella–zoster virus which is characterized by the appearance of spots and mild fever. It is passed on through airborne droplets and has an incubation period of between two and three weeks. The spots will form a rash, appearing in crops covering the trunk, arms, legs and face and can sometimes appear inside the mouth. The itchy spots turn into blisters which then dry out, leaving scabs. Once your child has had chickenpox, they are immune for life.

What you can do

Plenty of rest is the best treatment while your child has chickenpox. It is best to keep them away from other children for a couple of days from about a week after the spots appear, as this is when they are most contagious. To help prevent scratching, which can lead to scarring, apply soothing

Calamine lotion. Look out for signs of infection if your child can't stop scratching and contact your doctor if you have any doubts.

Treatment

Osteopathy An osteopath may use cranial work to help boost the immune system by decreasing mechanical strains and so enabling the release of more energy to fight off disease. This will also allow a better fluid interchange between tissues, for instance the blood and lymph.

Acupuncture Acupuncture can be of most value if given before the spots actually appear, in the first week or so after catching the disease, if possible. Chickenpox is seen as an accumulation of 'damp heat' trapped in the body, which erupts on the skin's surface in the form of pustules which seep pus and are itchy. An acupuncturist will treat the child to remove the heat from the surface and disperse the damp. The earlier treatment is given, the less likelihood there is of intense itchiness which can lead to scarring.

Aromatherapy An aromatherapist may recommend adding a few drops of oil, such as Lavender, Lemon and Geranium, to the child's bath to help relieve itching and to help prevent infection if they can't stop scratching. Lavender not only works as an antiseptic, but also helps skin tissue to regenerate. Lemon has properties which help to fight off infection and Geranium has astringent and anti-inflammatory qualities to help calm the skin.

Caution

Consult your doctor if there are signs that the spots have become infected, such as swelling, or if they haven't healed over. If, after about ten days, your child has fever, headaches and becomes clumsy – losing their balance – consult your doctor immediately as this may be a sign of encephalitis, or inflammation of the brain.

35

Other therapies that may be beneficial: homoeopathy, naturopathy.

CHILBLAINS

If your child is particularly sensitive to cold due to bad circulation, then chilblains may be a common occurrence. They are red, inflamed, itchy patches of skin, which are caused when the blood vessels near the surface of the skin narrow to keep in the heat in response to cold weather and then widen again when in the warmth. The skin tends to become pale and numb. Fingers, toes, ankles, ears and the backs of legs are most commonly affected. For some reason, girls tend to be more prone to chilblains than boys.

What you can do

Treatment is often not necessary, although putting talcum powder on the affected area may help to relieve the itching. Make sure your child is well wrapped up before going out in the cold.

Treatment

Traditional Chinese medicine If the problem is persistent, TCM may prove an effective therapy. A practitioner would see chilblains as a problem of yang deficiency. Herbal infusions including Ginger, Chinese Angelica and Red Sage, or Marigold may be used to help improve circulation.

Herbal medicine Dusting your child's feet with cayenne pepper mixed with talcum or arrowroot powder may help to keep them warm. A practitioner may advise a salve containing primrose leaves, lanolin, honey and thyme oil. Other treatments may include tincture of Myrrh, Rosemary, Lavender or Peppermint oil or Nettle juice. They may also suggest that your child could be lacking in calcium and silica which can be found in yoghurt, cheese, almonds, soybeans, lemon, and green vegetables.

Naturopathy A naturopath may recommend you give your child alternate warm and cool foot baths and that they only wear natural fibre shoes and socks. They may give mineral salt supplements such as calcium and iron phosphate or potassium chloride and vitamin B and E supplements to aid circulation. Ginger has properties which can help the circulation, so giving Ginger tea or increasing its intake in your child's food may be advised.

Aromatherapy If the skin is not feeling too sensitive then aromatherapy massage can help to bring relief to chilblains. Lemon can help the circulation while Sandalwood works well as an antiseptic. Foot baths containing a couple of drops of one of these oils can also be beneficial.

Other therapies that may be beneficial: reflexology, biochemic tissue salts.

COLD SORES

Facial cold sores are small blisters which form around the lips. They are usually preceded by a tingling sensation before the blisters appear. They can be sore and itchy until they burst and crust over, leaving a scab. They tend to last about a week. Cold sores are caused by the herpes simplex virus, and as they are highly contagious, most of the population carries the virus, having been infected at some point in their lives. Once infected, the virus will remain in the body, but stay dormant until re-activated, for instance by stress, exposure to cold or heat, or following an illness, when the immune system is low.

What you can do

Cold sores can be embarrassing for children – particularly teenagers – but you can help prevent your child getting recurrent attacks by avoiding known triggers, such as stressful situations, providing them with a well-balanced diet to help their immune system or wrapping a scarf around the lower part of their face in cold weather. Kissing should be avoided when the sores are present and the child should wash their hands after touching the affected area.

Treatment

Aromatherapy Applying Melissa (lemon balm) to the area where the first tingling signs warn of an oncoming sore can sometimes prevent the blisters forming. Use a fifty/fifty mix of Melissa with Grapeseed or Rosehip oil. An aromatherapist may use a mix of Geranium, Chamomile German, Lavender, Bergamot and Oregano, known for their antiviral properties, to help fight the condition as well as to reduce stress and anxiety which may trigger an attack.

Reflexology If your child suffers repeated attacks of the virus, reflexology works well in balancing the whole system, not just the area where the cold sore appears. Areas of the foot which may be worked on to help to reduce attacks, include those representing the endocrine, lymphatic and immune systems.

Traditional Chinese medicine This may combine acupuncture to help boost the immune system, as well as herbs. A diet of lots of grain and lightly cooked vegetables, avoiding dairy and sugary, fatty foods may also be advised. Cold sores are seen as a sign that the energy flow is blocked and the causes of this will need to be sought to help find relief.

Homoeopathy A homoeopath may choose remedies which will help to build up the child's constitution and boost the immune system to help prevent further attacks, as well as helping to reduce the pain and itchiness.

Other therapies that may be beneficial: naturopathy, Bach Flower Remedies, biochemic tissue salts, herbal medicine, acupuncture.

COLDS

There are around two hundred cold viruses and as these get passed on by sneezing or coughing or by being picked up by direct contact, it's not surprising that classrooms are ripe breeding grounds. There is no cure for the common cold. Once a child has become infected, the mucous membranes lining the nose and throat become inflamed, leading to a runny nose, sneezing, a sore throat and headaches. Other symptoms may include raised temperature, aching muscles and coughing. During a cold, the infection may spread from the throat to the middle ear, leading to ear ache and possibly on to glue ear. This is more likely in young children when the Eustachian tube is still small and therefore infection has less far to travel. (See also *Ear ache, Glue ear*.)

What you can do

Children can feel pretty miserable during a cold – they may be off their food, feel tired and irritable. Keep them warm and comfortable and offer plenty of fluids to prevent dehydration. If symptoms persist after a week, consult your doctor or practitioner in case of secondary infection or other underlying causes.

Treatment

Herbal medicine Herbal teas such as Fennel, Chamomile, and Lemon Balm should help relieve the symptoms of congestion and coughing. A practitioner may also recommend an infusion of Elderflower to help decongest, or Lime Flower to reduce mild fever. At home, sore throats may be eased by gargling with one part Myrrh to ten parts water.

Kinesiology A kinesiologist may detect a lowered endocrine and immune function, and apply various techniques accordingly to give the immune system a boost. A rotation diet with the right balance of foods, plenty of pure water and a reduction in sugar (which inhibits immune function) may be advised.

Traditional Chinese medicine The Chinese see a tendency to colds as 'wei qi xu' or a weakness of the protective energy and of the lungs. A doctor may prescribe jade screen powder, given from autumn onwards to help prevent repeated colds. Early on in the cold, the following 'tea' may help: 1oz (30g) of sliced root ginger, one broken-up cinnamon stick, one teaspoon (5ml) of coriander seeds, three cloves, one slice of lemon, all boiled in a pint (570ml) of water and simmered for ten minutes. Strain and give half a teacup every two hours. For children under three, one teaspoon (5ml) can be given every two hours.

Homoeopathy A homoeopath will concentrate on building up the child's immune system so that it can fight off future infection and treatment will depend on how the child is coping with the illness. A homoeopath may also recommend using the biochemic tissue salts such as Kali. mur. for catarrh, sore throat and wheezing and Kali. sulph. for the presence of mucus in the throat and nose.

Caution

Monitor your child for secondary infections if they are susceptible to bronchiolitis, bronchitis, asthma (see under relevant alphabetical section) or pneumonia.

Other therapies that may be beneficial: naturopathy, reflexology, homoeopathy, Bach Flower Remedies.

'Joe was a great newborn – a happy, placid, healthy child. But from about four months onwards, it all changed and he was constantly ill. He always had colds, hardly slept and was often constipated. I was at my wits' end because I was getting no sleep. He'd have maybe one day in three months when there wasn't something wrong with him. Looking back, the problems seemed to start after his four-month vaccinations. He was also circumcized at about that time. I took him to a homoeopath who told me that Joe had been through a lot of stressful events in his short life – birth, circumcision, immunization – and that being ill was his way of releasing stress. As he was still so small, a lot of the homoeopath's normal questions, such as Joe's likes and dislikes and so on, couldn't be answered. So he prescribed some pillules with about five or six remedies. Soon after, we got the first almost full night's sleep since he was born as Joe was breathing more easily. He's now three and the constipation continued to be a problem until recently. We discovered that rather than being constipated, every time we thought we saw Joe straining to let it all out he was actually straining to keep it all in. So now we've got to work on that problem.'

Gill and Joe, 3

COLIC

Many young babies suffer from colic which is thought to be caused by muscle spasms in the intestines or swallowed air, although no-one's sure why. Some doctors believe colic doesn't occur before one month, but there are many parents who would disagree. Symptoms include constant crying, with the legs being drawn up to the stomach, as if in pain, going red in the face and passing wind. It usually clears up at around twelve weeks. It is most common in the early evening but can go on for hours and can be distressing for parents to watch as well as being extremely exhausting to cope with.

What you can do

If normal soothing, such as walking around, rocking, feeding or burping don't seem to work, try bathing your baby around the worst time. This may distract them for a while as well as the warm water being comforting. Follow this by a gentle massage around the abdomen. Or placing a partially filled hand-warm hot-water bottle wrapped in a towel underneath their stomach may also be soothing. Keep reassuring your baby that you are close. If you are breastfeeding, watch your own diet – anything that irritates your stomach may irritate your baby's – so cut out foods such as cows' milk, strawberries, oranges, chocolate, spicy foods and coffee.

Treatment

Traditional Chinese medicine The Chinese see colic as a food blockage, stomach deficiency or cold. Acupuncture can sometimes bring immediate relief or a practitioner may advise an infusion of dill leaves or fennel seeds made up into a gripe water. TCM would also advise parents to leave two hours between feeds to prevent a food block, which may not be agreeable to mothers who feed on demand. For children under three with colic symptoms, the diet may be looked at as the Chinese believe too much wholefood can be too rough on the stomach.

Osteopathy Osteopaths believe that colic often arises as a result of a traumatic birth which has upset the cranial system. This in turn can affect the system which controls involuntary action such as gut and diaphragm movement, causing pain to the baby. By working on the cranial system, colic may be alleviated.

Chiropractic Chiropractic treatment of babies with colic has proved to be very helpful in many cases. Gentle manipulation of the midback and sometimes the upper neck will stimulate all of the nerves to the gut and can reduce colicky symptoms.

Homoeopathy A practitioner may advise giving Chamomilla if the baby is twisting in pain and is very irritable. Or, if the cramps seem severe and are accompanied by diarrhoea and flatulence, Nux Vomica. If the abdomen is very tight and the abdomen distended, Mag. Carb.

'My son Jonah was three weeks old when he had his first session of cranial osteopathy. I'd read about it and knew that for colic the sooner you started treatment, the better the results. Liz, the osteopath would pop round to my house once a week for sessions.

'I knew of some mothers who said their baby's colic disappeared after only one go, but Jonah being Jonah, he took five. Liz said she could work better if the baby was asleep, but Jonah always managed to be wide awake when she turned up, which is why I think treatment took longer. He was a very restless, discontented baby and during the evenings wouldn't stop crying and arching his body away from us, no matter what we tried to do to soothe him.

'There wasn't much improvement after the first session and as Liz seemed to be only holding him, I began to wonder what my £25 was being spent on. But after the second time, he had definitely improved. By the end of the fifth, he was a completely different baby – contented, relaxed and free from pain. Now he's the most laid back, placid toddler who's always got a smile on his face!'

Pippa and Jonah, now a toddler

CONJUNCTIVITIS

This is a common complaint in children as it is infectious and is easily passed on through hand-to-eye contact. Bacterial or viral infections such as a sore throat causes the conjunctiva membrane of the eye to become inflamed and itchy, discharging a yellow pus. On waking in the morning, the child may find their eyelids crusty and stuck together. Conjunctivitis can also be caused by an allergy, for instance from pollen or to chemicals used in swimming pools. (See *Allergies*). Newborn babies can suffer a form of conjunctivitis which blocks the tear ducts soon after birth if they develop an infection from the mother's cervix. In more serious cases, this can lead to blindness, so medical treatment should be sought immediately.

What you can do
Gently swabbing the eye with cotton wool dipped in warm, sterilized water or breast milk will help clear the ducts and wipe away crusts. If both eyes are infected, swab each eye with a clean ball of cotton wool. Give your child a separate flannel and towel to help prevent the spread of infection. Keep their hands as clean as possible and try to discourage them from touching their eyes.

Treatment
Naturopathy A naturopath will see the appearance of conjunctivitis as a sign that the immune system is weakened. To boost this, they may recommend foods rich in vitamins A, C and E and zinc, found in fruit and vegetables. They may also advise mineral salt supplements which help to support the body's system, such as potassium chloride, or iron and magnesium phosphate. The eye may also be bathed in cooled Eyebright tea or a cup of saline solution also containing a drop of Golden Seal.

Herbal medicine An eyewash using Eyebright, Raspberry or Calendula will help to soothe the eye and clear infection. Or Eyebright, made into a compress with cotton wool or gauze and applied to the eye for fifteen minutes, or even drunk in an infusion, may be recommended.

Osteopathy Sometimes where there is restrictive movement

in the facial bones, the eye cannot drain properly. An osteopath may gently try to manipulate the bones to help alleviate the problem.

Homoeopathy A homoeopath might recommend Aconite if the condition is due to exposure to cold. If there is a lot of discharge, Argentium nit. may be advised.

Caution

See your GP or practitioner if symptoms do not clear up within twenty-four hours.

CONSTIPATION

Bowel actions vary from child to child and although one child might only go every three days, while another twice a day, both can be seen as normal, as long as they are regular. But when bowel movement becomes irregular and the stools are dry, hard and difficult to pass, it is a sign of constipation. Causes can include lack of fibre, lack of fluids or essential fatty acids. Fibre-rich foods such as wholegrains, cereals, potatoes, vegetables and fruit are all needed to keep the bowels healthy. Essential fatty acids are found in oily fish, oils such as rape seed, and nuts like walnuts (although children under seven should not be given nuts). If stools are difficult to pass, your child may be afraid to go to the loo, prolonging the problem. Children whose parents have tried to force bowel movements in an attempt to form regularity may find that the child reacts by holding back.

What you can do

Make sure your child has a diet high in fibre and drinks plenty of fluids to keep the bowel moving and stools soft. Giving them dried fruit, such as apricots or prunes, to chew on instead of sweets should help, too. Don't pressurize them into going or try to hurry them along.

Treatment

Hypnotherapy Some therapists may put the child into a trance and tell them they are no longer to be constipated. Or they may be analysed to find the reason for the 'holding in', to find the cause of the problem, in the belief that this in itself will solve the problem. But, more popularly, a hypnotherapist may help a child, who for instance feels disgust at passing stools, to disassociate the negative feelings at going to the loo and use the feelings in a more positive way so that holding in is no longer necessary.

Naturopathy The naturopath will check the child's toileting history, asking questions like 'are they worried about germs' and 'do they see the toilet as a nasty place to be?' If so, it may help to make the bathroom a cheerful and relaxed place to be, with books and toys, although they should not be encouraged to sit for too long. It will also be advised that their intake of water is increased, that they get plenty of fibre from fruit and vegetables and well-cooked whole grains, but that they avoid bran which can irritate the bowel and decreases the absorption of calcium, magnesium and the B vitamins. Linseeds, which have been soaked daily, will help to soothe the bowel and make the passage of the stools easier. Exercise will be encouraged. It may also help to reintroduce a potty for a young child as this gives a more natural squatting position for opening the bowels.

Acupuncture Acupuncturists see constipation as often being caused by heat in the body. With a lack of body fluids the stools will be small and dry. They will check whether the reason for the constipation is that the constitution is weak and that therefore there is not enough Qi or energy flow for normal bodily functions. Or whether the patient is strong, but eating the wrong types of food and not taking in enough fluids in between meals, so that not enough mucus is produced to aid the passing of stools. Acupuncturists also believe that seasonal changes may be a factor.

Osteopathy Osteopaths believe that constipation can be the result of a spinal and/or pelvic imbalance, so that the nerve and blood supplies to the bowel may be affected. They will work to restore these imbalances and restore bowel function. In newborn babies, a traumatic birth can lead to constipation, and cranial work has shown results within seconds!

Caution

If constipation continues, despite a good diet, or blood appears when stools are passed, consult a doctor.

COUGH

Coughing is a reflex action to try and rid the throat of any irritant or blockages. This can be due to mucus build-up after an infection, exposure to cigarette smoke or due to an allergy, for instance to pollen. Coughs can be a sign of a more severe problem such as croup, bronchitis (see under relevant alphabetical section) or pneumonia.

What you can do

Coughs shouldn't be suppressed, unless you have been advised otherwise, as they help to clear phlegm from the airways. Propping your child up at night may make breathing easier. Gentle patting on the back during a coughing attack may help to loosen phlegm. A hot drink of water, lemon and honey can help to soothe a throat that has become sore after coughing. Avoid smoking in any of the rooms that your child uses.

Treatment

Naturopathy A naturopath will aim to boost the immune system, which may have been weakened due to illness, by suggesting an increase in foods rich in vitamins A, C, E and zinc, such as fruit and vegetables. Onions, garlic and honey will help too. It may also help to cut back on foods that produce mucus, such as dairy products and sweets. Mineral salts, which help to support the system, may also be given, but the choice will depend on whether the cough is acute or chronic as well as seeing which other symptoms are present. A tepid pack put on the chest or alternating a hot and cold compress on the chest may help to loosen phlegm. Herbal remedies such as Comfrey, Wild Cherry Bark, Coltsfoot, Echinacea and Golden Seal may also be given.

Herbal medicine Treatment will depend on the child. But a practitioner may recommend herbs such as Marsh Mallow, Hyssop and Eucalyptus. Garlic, known for its qualities in helping coughs, colds and chesty ailments, may also be given. It can be taken fresh in food, or in capsules or tincture.

Aromatherapy Massage using aromatherapy oils can help to loosen phlegm. A therapist may advise an inhalation to help with the mucus, such as two drops each of Eucalyptus, Sandalwood and Bergamot, dropped into a bowl of near-boiling water (hold firmly to prevent spillage, and protect the child's chest with thick towels). Place a towel over the child's head and encourage them to breathe deeply. Asthmatic children should avoid doing this. Alternatively, sprinkle a couple of drops of one of the oils on to their handkerchief to inhale.

Homoeopathy If your child's cough is short and dry, accompanied by a raised temperature, a homoeopath may recommend Aconite. For a watery or bubbly cough, Ars. alb. may be prescribed, or Rumex crispus for a tickly throat that leads to coughing.

Biochemic tissue salts Ferr. phos. may be used for a dry cough and raised temperature, or if the cough is worse at night, Kali. sulph. There are combination packs specifically for coughs and colds, such as Combination J or Q.

'Sophie first started getting a cough when she was two. As soon as she laid down when I put her to bed, she'd start coughing and it would go on all night. She'd cough so much her stomach muscles would hurt with the strain. I took her to my GP who said she had asthma – and immediately prescribed antibiotics and Ventolin. But I wasn't convinced that that was the problem or happy with her taking such drugs when she was so young.

'So although I took the prescription, I decided to try herbs. The practitioner asked lots of questions about our family background, Sophie's health, what she ate and so on and listened to Sophie coughing. She then said Sophie didn't have asthma at all. Her tonsils are just very large and swollen and sensitive to any triggers such as smoke. This made her cough and was aggravated by colds. She was given a herbal tea to drink three times a day which doesn't taste too good, so she takes it in one gulp. The practitioner also suggested gargling with a weak salt solution as Sophie's not great at brushing her teeth and the bacteria in her mouth could be irritating her tonsils. The difference is amazing – she hasn't coughed since and we all get to sleep.'

Jill and Sophie, 6

CRADLE CAP

The presence of thick, greasy yellow scales on patches of the scalp, known as cradle cap, is quite common in babies. It can also cover the face, neck and behind the ears, which all tend to produce more oil than other areas. It is a form of dermatitis which can recur and, although not usually a problem, it is very noticeable on some babies and can look a little unsightly.

What you can do

Although treatment is not often necessary, you can wash your baby's hair with a mild shampoo and gently rub in an oil such as olive every day to help loosen the scales. Regular brushing will also help the scales to break away.

Treatment

Herbal medicine For persistent cradle cap, apply Calendula cream which works particularly well for skin problems, to help soften the flakes so they are more easily removed.

Aromatherapy For dry patches, such as behind the ears, gently massage in one drop of Rose or Lavender mixed with 50ml of almond oil.

CROUP

Croup is a dry, barking cough that can come on quite suddenly, usually in young children. The sound is caused by air passing through the narrowed, inflamed airways. Younger children are particularly susceptible as their bronchi, or air passages, are still small and more easily blocked with mucus. The child may also have a raised temperature, and be restless. Croup tends to occur after an infection, such as bronchitis, but can be due to an allergy.

What you can do

An attack may last for up to twelve hours, but won't necessarily need treatment. In winter, it will help to put bowls of water near hot radiators to help humidify the room. Stay close to your child, calming them so they don't panic and make breathing more difficult. Support them with pillows to raise the chest and facilitate breathing in bed. If your child is struggling for breath, or beginning to turn blue, call medical help immediately.

Treatment

Naturopathy Cutting down on foods that increase the production of mucus, such as dairy products, may be advised. Sticking to organic foods and taking vitamin supplements suitable for children may also be recommended to help build up the body's immunity. Mineral salt supplements may be given, such as calcium and iron phosphate and potassium chloride to help support the body. It may also be advisable to turn off the central heating in the child's room, which can dry out the air.

Hydrotherapy Moist, damp air will help ease croup. Take your child into the bathroom, and run the hot bath and sink taps to create a humid atmosphere which will help them breathe more easily.

Homoeopathy A practitioner may start by prescribing Aconite for the dry bark, followed by Spongia if there is no improvement. Drosera might also be recommended for a tickly cough that is worse at night.

Caution

Call for medical help if your child is having breathing difficulties.

CRYING

All children cry, but sometimes it may be hard to understand why or you may just feel there is more to your child being upset than meets the eye. In babies, although the reasons are usually more obvious, you may not be able to see anything wrong and yet your child is trying to tell you that all is not right. They may just need comfort, they may be hungry, or if colic is bothering them, need a remedy to relieve it (see *Colic*). But if the crying is persistent and means broken sleep for nights on end, it can be very distressing for both parent and baby. As they grow up, there may be more complex reasons for bouts of crying. Young children may find a new sibling threatening and need more attention, finding crying the only way to get it, or it may be a signal of some internal problem, such as a stomach or ear ache. Older children may

have problems with playmates or at school and need an outlet at home for their unhappiness.

What you can do

In babies, plenty of comfort and attention may be all that's
needed and it may take trying many different positions before
you find one that soothes. But relentless crying can be very
wearing, so if you're a new parent, nap when you can during
the day. Desperate parents have been known to take mid-
night car drives in order for the engine sound and movement
to lull their baby to sleep. Try to talk to older children about
their crying. If it's more than a physical problem, it may take
time for the real reason for their distress to become apparent.

Treatment

Hypnotherapy A hypnotherapist may help the child to use
their inner resources – times when they were contented and
happy and had no need to cry – and learn to apply those
resources to times in their lives when they need them.

Herbal medicine If you are feeling concerned or distressed by
your baby's crying, there are a number of herbs that have a
calming effect. Lavender, Chamomile, Lemon Balm, Hops
and Catmint all have soothing properties and can be given in
diluted cool teas before bedtime or if the baby wakes during
the night.

Osteopathy Osteopaths believe that the process of birth is
traumatic for a baby, particularly if it was a difficult birth. This
can affect the baby's cranial system, which will be worked on.
Once any problems have been corrected, the baby hopefully
stops crying.

CUTS/GRAZES

Minor cuts, grazes and scratches are harmless, as long as an
infection doesn't set in, and should heal well on their own.

What you can do

If needed, apply light pressure to stop the bleeding. Clean well with water and ensure the area is kept clean and dry. Apply bandaging, if necessary.

Treatment

Aromatherapy Apply a drop of Tea-Tree or Lavender oil diluted in an egg-cup full of tepid water and dab on the cut. Geranium, Lavender, Eucalyptus, Lemon and Pine are also useful to help promote healing and prevent infection setting in.

Homoeopathy Calendula lotion or ointment applied to the cut will help soothe. If the child has suffered a little shock Arnica will have a calming effect. If the wound has become infected, a homoeopath may recommend Hepar. sulph.

Bach Flower Remedies Rescue Cream, which is a lanolin-free cream containing six flower remedies, works well for minor cuts and grazes. After cleaning the skin, apply the cream to the affected area and repeat, as necessary.

Biochemic tissue salts If the cut or graze is slow to heal, Calc. sulph. may help speed up the process.

CYSTITIS

Not just a problem for adults, children suffer from cystitis too. Cystitis is an infection of the bladder. It may be caused by an infection due to the backflow of urine. Or if the child has been on a course of antibiotics, this may result in the yeast infection, thrush, which can also lead on to an infection. If your child is suffering from constipation, this may add to the problem. As with adults, this can become a continual problem as antibiotics are given for the cystitis, which can cause an imbalance of bacteria, leading to the growth of thrush and then more susceptibility to infection, leading again to cystitis.

Symptoms may include a constant need to go to the loo, although in many children the only symptoms will be pain when passing urine and a raised temperature.

What you can do

Encourage your child to drink plenty of fluids. Concentrated urine will be more irritable to pass. It will also help to frequently flush bacteria out of the body. They should always pass urine as soon as possible when they feel the need and completely empty their bladder. Don't use bubble baths or talcum powder while the infection is present as this may just irritate further. Make sure they know to wipe from front to back, to avoid spreading any infection from the anal area. After urinating or passing stools, the area should be wiped (front to back) with warm water and then patted dry.

Treatment

Naturopathy Cranberry juice, particularly during an attack of cystitis, is thought to be beneficial as research has shown it prevents bacteria from clinging to the bladder walls. However, it is very tart and many consumer brands are high in sugar to counteract this. An unsweetened cranberry extract tablet may be a good alternative. Blueberries also seem to be beneficial in a similar way. A naturopath may recommend increasing your child's water intake to two pints (1 litre) a day. The naturopath will also look at your child's diet as a sensitivity to some foods is also thought to play a part. Tea, coffee, sugar, orange juice, vinegar, spice, dairy products and gluten can all be culprits. And if your child also suffers from thrush, foods containing yeast or mould, such as bread, mushrooms and blue cheese may also need to be eliminated. If your child gets into a cycle of cystitis followed by thrush, natural live yoghurt or the supplement acidophilus and bifidus should restore the balance of bacteria in the gut.

Herbal medicine For chronic cystitis, homemade lemon barley water may help to bring relief. One herbal remedy is to boil one tablespoon (15ml) of pearl barley in two cups (450ml) of water for twenty minutes, strain, cool and add one teaspoon (5ml) of fresh lemon juice. Give to your child to drink twice a day. Or a decoction of Couchgrass and Horsetail may also help to bring relief. Couchgrass contains properties which help to soothe irritation and inflammation and is particularly useful for urinary tract infections. Horsetail acts as an astringent and will help to heal.

Acupuncture An acupuncturist may see cystitis as damp and cold pervading the outer layers of the body's defensive Qi or vital energy. This 'cold' then turns to heat in the body, causing the bladder to become inflamed and cause irritation during urination. Although conventional antibiotics can reduce the heat and infection in the short term, the problem returns whenever the child is in a similar situation to the one that first caused the problem. The acupuncturist would work on certain points to remove the localized inflammation and then treat the root cause to prevent recurrence.

Osteopathy Tension in the spine and in local soft tissue can affect the functioning of the kidneys. The osteopath will work to correct these and any problems that predisposed the cystitis to occur.

Other therapies that may be beneficial: reflexology, traditional Chinese medicine.

'I used to be a real non-believer when it came to herbal medicine, but when my daughter became so ill, my mum, who's been using it for years, persuaded me to try it. I thought it would be a waste of money, but I was desperate.

'Joanne was always suffering from tonsillitis. She'd have a course of antibiotics to clear it, but then the next month she'd have

---

to have more when the tonsillitis came back. She would get cystitis as a result as her immune system became weakened and she built up resistance to the drugs, so infection spread easily. It got so bad the infection spread to her kidneys and she had to be hospitalized. They eventually took her tonsils out and she didn't need antibiotics anymore, but the cystitis still kept returning. She'd scream with pain when she went to the loo, but the doctors said there was nothing they could do to prevent it, just treat it.

'So I made an appointment to see a herbalist. She took details of Joanne's family and medical history and gave her a small bottle of herbs to take with cranberry juice. Within hours, the pain had gone. Even the herbalist was surprised it had worked so quickly.

'When we went for our appointment, the herbs were changed slightly. She got one more bout of cystitis, but since then has been totally well.'

Lorraine and Joanne, 7

DIARRHOEA

The occasional bout of diarrhoea can be due to a number of causes, the most common being gastroenteritis caused by a viral or bacterial infection from contaminated food. Other causes can be food intolerance, a reaction to drugs, such as antibiotics, or something that has disagreed with them. The small intestine lining becomes damaged, so that food passes through without the usual amount of water being absorbed, leading to a 'runny tummy'. In babies and young children, diarrhoea can be very serious because of the risk of rapid dehydration, especially if accompanied with vomiting. Sometimes diarrhoea can be a symptom of another problem such as stress or nerves.

What you can do

In moderately severe diarrhoea, try to avoid giving a baby milk (except breast milk) until the diarrhoea starts to settle. Give instead an electrolyte mixture, which can be bought ready prepared from chemists and which will help restore the body's lost water and salts. Alternatively, give a cup of water with a pinch of salt and one teaspoon (5ml) of sugar. You can also give small sips of water or very diluted juice. In young children milk can be gradually reintroduced once the diarrhoea begins to improve. Avoid apple juice, as this can trigger the condition.

Treatment

Medical attention should be sought, but the following complementary therapies may also be beneficial:

Homoeopathy A homoeopath may prescribe Baptisia for 'flu-like symptoms and gastritis and Belladonna, if accompanied by a raised temperature. If the diarrhoea is due to a stress-related problem for the child, Gelsemium may be used, or Borax if the child is particularly nervous.

Acupuncture An acupuncturist would look at a number of possible causes of the diarrhoea. It may be due to overeating or irregular eating, particularly of foods seen as having a 'cold' influence, or different types of weather, such as damp or summer heat, may have an effect. Illness and the use of antibiotics can affect the bowel. Or the child may have a weak constitution or have had a severe illness. Depending on what the acupuncturist sees as the cause, treatment will vary, to make up for deficiencies, for instance in the stomach and spleen.

Naturopathy Diarrhoea more often occurs in bottlefed rather than breastfed babies. Give water rather than a bottle for twenty-four hours, while monitoring closely for signs of dehydration. If a breastfed baby has diarrhoea, the mother should look at her own diet for the cause, as it may be a sign

of allergy to certain foods. If an older child is prone to diarrhoea, a close look at their diet may be necessary. A naturopath will advise that suppressants should not be used, as
diarrhoea is the body's natural way of eliminating unwanted
waste. Fluids should be kept up – taking regular sips every
twenty minutes or so. A gradual return to solids, keeping
foods simple such as white toast, green apples without their
skin and bananas (remove the central vein), is best.
Supplements and mineral salts such as potassium chloride,
sodium sulphate and iron phosphate may be recommended.

Kinesiology A test will be carried out to check for an imbalance in the bowel, for instance after a stomach bug. Various
points may be rubbed to correct the imbalance and relieve
any uncomfortable symptoms.

Caution

Call for medical help immediately if a baby or young child
shows signs of dehydration following diarrhoea. Symptoms
include drowsiness, lethargy, lack of response, glazed eyes,
persistent crying, a depressed fontanelle, loose skin. A doctor
should also be called if diarrhoea persists for more than six
hours. Serious cases may need hospital treatment with intravenous fluids.

'Chris, who's two, had had diarrhoea for a couple of days. I took
him to an acupuncturist because I'd tried acupuncture myself in
the past and I also knew that it could work more quickly than
some other therapies. I wasn't apprehensive about the needles,
as I knew there would be just a little tingling feeling and that I'd
be close by if Chris didn't like it.

'The acupuncturist asked a lot of questions about Chris. Two
of the main things that emerged were that Chris had just found a
new playmate who he spent a lot of time with, so was getting

very over-tired which could have been contributory, and that I'd just switched from giving him orange juice to apple juice. I was told that apples have a very cooling effect on the stomach, which can lead to diarrhoea. After just one session and switching juices, his diarrhoea was gone.

'At the same time, both my children were starting to get little patches of eczema. I was taught how to put finger pressure on points above and beside each kneecap and elbow for three minutes. Every day the kids would remind me, "got to do our points, mummy". Because it was only mild eczema and we started early, it was gone in a week.

'It feels so good to be in control of my children's health, rather than being handed out a prescription.'

Sue and Chris, 2

EAR ACHE (*otitis media*)

Ear ache is very common in children, particularly acute *otitis media* which is infection of the middle ear. Younger children suffer more as the Eustachian tube, which connects the ear to the nose and throat, is still short and infection spreads more easily. Other causes may be toothache, tonsillitis, mumps (see under relevant alphabetical section) or infection of the outer ear (*otitis externa*), such as a boil. Occasionally, the cause may be due to something such as an insect entering the ear. Ear ache causes a sharp, stabbing pain and may be accompanied by a discharge of pus, raised temperature and slight loss of hearing due to a build-up of fluid in the ear. Babies with ear ache may signal discomfort by pulling or scratching at their ear.

What you can do

Don't try to stick anything down a child's ear as this may push any foreign body or wax further down. Check the child's temperature. Keep them warm and comfortable – placing a wrapped-up hot-water bottle on their pillow will soothe – and take care when washing so water doesn't enter the ear.

Treatment

Acupressure If the ear ache is due to a cold or a change in pressure, such as during air travel, try pressure with two or three fingers (depending on how big the child is) on the area in front of the ears for two or three minutes.

Naturopathy A naturopath may suggest that frequent ear ache may be due to a diet too high in mucus-forming foods, such as dairy products. If antibiotics have been given previously, the child's immunity may be lowered and probiotics, such as acidophilus and bifidus, may be recommended to rebalance. A diet containing plenty of foods containing vitamins A as beta carotene, C, E and zinc may be recommended. The herbal remedy Muellin oil might be given, as a few drops into the ear every few hours can bring pain relief, or Lavender oil, rubbed behind the ears, may be advised.

Reflexology All the toes would be worked on which correlate to the head, but particularly at the ear point found at the base of the fourth and fifth toes which relates to the Eustachian tube. Other parts of the body may also be treated, such as the intestine, to help promote overall health.

Homoeopathy If the child becomes very sensitive to noise and has a raised temperature, a homoeopath may recommend Aconite or Belladonna for the acute, throbbing and pain associated with ear ache. Chamomilla may be given to soothe the pain when the face is red and the child distressed.

Biochemic tissue salts For an acute attack, Ferr. phos. may work well. If there is a slight discharge from the ear, Calc. phos. may be recommended.

Caution

Ear ache can lead to more severe problems such as glue ear

(see under *Glue ear*) or may affect hearing, so consult a doctor at the first signs.
Other therapies that may be beneficial: osteopathy, chiropractic, aromatherapy.

'My two children have always been cared for through naturopathy. They've rarely been sick and have never needed antibiotics. If they do get ill then I decide which is the best way to treat them. So when Sam had an ear infection, I made up a herbal infusion to give as ear drops. He lets everyone know when he's sick, so I knew it had cleared up within two or three hours. If it had not got any better within twelve hours then I would have taken him to the doctor.

'Sam and Joe eat very healthily which is why they're not often ill. I give them lots of organic fruit and vegetables and avoid processed food. Sam was breastfed until he was eighteen months old, didn't have solids until he was seven months and wasn't given dairy produce until he was two-and-a-half. Even so, he's sensitive to dairy and I try to avoid giving it to him. If he gets a cough or cold, I'll give him a herbal remedy and make sure he gets plenty of rest and he tends to recover quite quickly.'

Jaine (naturopath) and Sam, 5 and Joe, 18 months

ECZEMA

Atopic eczema is common in children and although it tends not to affect newborns, very occasionally some children are born with the condition. In the areas affected, such as the face, hands, armpits, elbows and groin area, the skin becomes inflamed, scaly and itchy and sometimes blisters form. The cause isn't always known, but it often occurs as an allergic reaction and sometimes following immunization. It does tend to run in families with a history of asthma and rhinitis, or it can be linked to stress. Many susceptible babies suffer an attack when first introduced to solids. Children tend to grow out of this type of eczema as they reach adolescence.

What you can do

Stick to cotton clothing for your child and prevent them from becoming overheated, as this may make the eczema more itchy. Minimize contact with possible allergens, such as certain foods if you think these may be a problem, pets, biological soap powders, down pillows and duvets (see *Allergies*). Use a gentle emollient cream to help prevent the skin from drying out.

Treatment

Naturopathy A naturopath will make a detailed study of your child's habit and lifestyle to determine possible causes of the eczema. They will then make recommendations to adapt that lifestyle and detoxify the body. This may include avoiding foods the body believes are toxic and may be allergic to, such as dairy, additives and colourings, wheat, soya and sugar. Herbal medicine may also be used to help with the detoxification. A herbal skin cream will also help to give temporary relief. Mineral salt supplements may also be recommended to help support the system, such as potassium sulphate and calcium or sodium phosphate.

Kinesiology The practitioner will check to see if there are any bowel or hydration problems which may be causing blockages and if there are any nutritional deficiencies. As emotions can play a major part in triggering eczema, possible stress factors for the child will be looked for and worked on. Angry, itchy eczema can be quickly relieved, but until the necessary lifestyle changes are made, it may take a while to disappear completely.

Traditional Chinese medicine There have been some positive studies into the use of Chinese herbs and eczema. One study, continued in a follow-up survey, revealed positive results, with eighteen of the thirty-seven children monitored having 90 per cent reductions in eczema. By the end of the year-long study, seven children discontinued treatment without relapsing. The practitioner will assess the child as a whole and will take into account their diet and lifestyle as well as the problem itself. Acupuncture (see below) to relieve the blocked meridians may be given, as well as doses of herbs, made up for the individual, to help resolve the problem of damp heat or dryness.

Acupuncture Acupuncturists see eczema as a symptom rather than a cause. They believe it is associated with three types of heat: damp heat, where the skin is itchy, hot and weeping; dry heat, where the skin is dry, red and itchy; and wind heat, when the skin breaks out and forms scabs, coming and going from different parts of the body. Treatment will depend on the child's type of eczema according to these forms.

Caution

Do not exclude foods from your child's diet without first consulting your practitioner or doctor.

Other therapies that may be beneficial: hypnotherapy, reflexology, aromatherapy, homoeopathy, herbal medicine, osteopathy.

'Gemma was born with eczema, which is quite unusual. It covered her whole body, but was particularly bad on her head and face. Things got worse when she was about four months old. She got chickenpox, so as well as eczema, her body was covered in spots. The illness weakened her a lot and as a result her skin became even worse. It got so bad she was sent to a paediatric dermatologist at Great Ormond Street Hospital for Sick

Children in London. Each night we had to smear Vaseline containing steroids on Gemma's body and then cover her up with damp bandages followed by dry ones. But that didn't work and when they suggested oral steroids, we really felt we wanted to try something else.

'So the hospital referred me to a Chinese doctor who has a clinic there. Gemma was given a large dose of a whole blend of herbs which were brewed into a tea. We just mixed this into her drinks and the taste didn't seem to bother her. The difference was astonishing. Her eczema improved almost immediately, but after about six to eight weeks the change was dramatic.

'Now we just take her every five weeks for a check-up and the herbs are altered according to how she is.'

John and Gemma, 3

FEVER (raised temperature)

If your child has a raised temperature, or fever, it may be a symptom of a cold or 'flu or a more serious illness, such as tonsillitis, chickenpox, middle ear infection or measles. A normal temperature is between 36° and 37°C (96.8–98.6°F) and fever is defined as over 37°C. A fever may be accompanied with other symptoms, depending on the cause of the illness, such as headache, drowsiness, rapid breathing, sweating, irritability, flushed face and shivering. A fever is serious in a young baby, particularly in those under six months, as it may cause febrile convulsions, when the baby will twitch or jerk and lose consciousness for a few minutes.

What you can do

Monitor your child's temperature regularly if they have a fever. Keep them in a cool room and cover with as little as possible. Sponge down your child all over with tepid (not cold) water, until their temperature begins to fall. Give plenty of fluids to drink. Don't give aspirin unless advised by a doctor. Let the child sleep as much as they want to.

Treatment

Herbal medicine Herbal medicine sees fever as the body's way of expelling, so it is a perfectly natural function that should not be suppressed. But Elderflowers may be recommended to help with the fever and are also a useful natural laxative. Yarrow is also known to help the body deal with fever and Lime Blossom has properties which will help any sweating and also relax the child. A herbalist may also recommend giving one teaspoon (5ml) of cider vinegar in a cup of water, to be sipped throughout the day.

Bach Flower Remedies There are a number of remedies that may be recommended, depending on the personality of the child and how they feel about being ill. Crab Apple has a cleansing effect and so is useful after any illness to help purify the body and get rid of the feeling of sickness. If the child is lacking energy after being ill, Olive may help the child to return to normal by helping to restore strength and vitality.

Homoeopathy If the temperature rises suddenly, and the child is very thirsty and has hot skin, Belladonna may be recommended. If the baby seems very fidgety and restless and is worse late at night, Arsenicum may be useful. If movement causes the baby distress and large amounts of fluid are being drunk, Bryonia may also be useful.

Biochemic tissue salts A homoeopath or other practitioner may also recommend the use of tissue salts for fever. Ferr. phos. is thought to help with symptoms. Kali mur. may also be advised for any accompanying catarrh or cold.

Caution

If your baby suffers a convulsion, call your doctor immediately.

Other therapies that may be beneficial: reflexology, aromatherapy.

FOOD POISONING

Food poisoning is caused by eating contaminated food. This can be food that has not been cooked properly or thoroughly defrosted, or contains bacteria passed on by hands that have not been washed before handling the food. Symptoms, which usually appear after between one and forty-eight hours, include stomach cramps, diarrhoea, raised temperature, loss of appetite and vomiting. The most common bacterium are salmonella (found in poultry, eggs and egg products such as mayonnaise), campylobacter (found in unpasteurized milk and cheese and in poor hygienic conditions), listeria (found in soft and blue cheeses, some types of pâté and cook-chill and ready-to-eat meals), and E. coli, which can cause poisoning in babies who have drunk from unsterilized or poorly sterilized bottles. Foods that have been in water contaminated with human excrement, such as shellfish, can also be a cause. Children can also be poisoned by eating poisonous plants or fungi.

Food poisoning is serious in babies as the accompanying symptoms of vomiting and diarrhoea can lead to dehydration and, in severe cases, be fatal.

What you can do

Make sure your child drinks plenty of fluids, but avoids solids. To prevent dehydration, give rehydration solutions containing salt and glucose. These can be bought from chemists, or you can make up your own, by mixing one level teaspoon (5ml) of salt and eight level teaspoons (40ml) of sugar to two pints (one litre) of cooled boiled water, to be drunk throughout the day. Get rid of any foods that you feel may be the cause of the food poisoning. Slowly reintroduce simple solid foods, such as soups and bananas or plain rice and avoid milk until symptoms have eased.

For future prevention you should always:

- wash your hands before handling food and after handling raw meat
- rinse fresh fruit and vegetables before cooking and eating
- use a separate chopping board for cutting meat
- thoroughly defrost food before cooking
- thoroughly cook or reheat any meals, particularly those containing meat
- refrigerate all cooked food and check your fridge is cold enough (below 10°C).

Treatment
*Medical attention should be sought, but the following comple-
mentary therapies may also be beneficial:*
Homoeopathy A practitioner may prescribe Bryonia for the vomiting and diarrhoea and if the child feels discomfort with every movement. If the child is feeling particularly weak and is suffering from vomiting and diarrhoea, especially at night, China may be prescribed. If a baby feels cold and restless and obviously unwell, Arsenicum may be advised.

Traditional Chinese medicine Treatment will depend on the type of poisoning. If it is as a result of seafood poisoning, ginger, Chinese olive and reed grass may be prescribed. For fighting against the types of bacteria found in improperly defrosted, undercooked food or in unhygienic conditions Mishmi bitter may be used. Garlic may also be recommended. Chinese 'Pochai pills' may be given to deal with the food poisoning and food stagnation.

Naturopathy A naturopath would recommend avoiding all solid food until the symptoms had eased and that the child sip at least one to two pints (½ to 1 litre) of water a day. Ginger tea may also help to calm the stomach. Once the symptoms have eased, dry white toast may be nibbled. Then more solid, but simple food can be slowly introduced such as brown rice or some fruit or vegetables. To help give support, mineral salt supplements may be recommended, such as potassium chloride, iron and magnesium phosphate and sodium sulphate. After vomiting, your child's natural balance of bacteria in the gut may be disturbed, so a probiotic supplement such as acidophilus and bifidus may be recommended or that you give your child live yoghurt which contains bacteria necessary for the bowel.

Caution

If your baby has been suffering from diarrhoea and vomiting for more than six hours, seek medical attention to prevent dehydration.

GLUE EAR

Glue ear is quite common in children and occurs when fluid accumulates in the middle ear cavity, usually when there is catarrh, associated with a viral infection such as a cold, tonsillitis or enlarged adenoids. The Eustachian tube, which runs from the ear to the throat, becomes blocked, so the fluid is unable to drain away. Eventually, pressure may lead the ear drum to burst. Both ears tend to be affected and the blockage affects the sound vibrations, leading to impaired hearing. This can sometimes go undetected and the child begins to have trouble hearing at school, which may lead to inattention, and both teachers and parents can wrongly believe the child is being difficult or unresponsive.

What you can do

It is thought there may be a connection between children who are bottlefed and glue ear, as the action of breastfeeding exercises the muscle that helps to open the Eustachian tube, which bottlefeeding does not do.

If your child is showing signs of irritability or vagueness when listening to you, or teachers complain of sudden inattentiveness at school, check whether your child may have an ear blockage. If you think your child has hearing problems, consult a doctor or practitioner as soon as possible. Early detection may mean avoiding more serious treatment, such as the insertion of grommets – small plastic tubes – which are placed in the ear by an ear, nose and throat specialist under general anaesthetic, allowing the mucus to drain away. These fall out once the problem has cleared up or are removed. Underlying causes such as adenoids or tonsils may need to be removed to prevent persistent recurrences.

It's better not to let babies have bottles while lying down, as this increases the risk of fluid draining into the ear and then becoming infected. Try to always hold and support a feeding child.

Treatment

Herbal medicine Echinacea, Wild Indigo and Elderflower will help to halt the infection, improve the child's immune system and help dry up the mucus. If the eardrum hasn't burst, infused oils of Hypericum mixed with a few drops of Eucalyptus may help reduce the inflammation.

Naturopathy The child's diet will be analysed and as allergy to dairy produce, wheat or soya may increase the amount of mucus produced, these may need to be avoided and substituted. Eating garlic, onions and chillies may help to reduce mucus. Mullein oil may be prescribed to ease congestion. Mineral salts may be given, to help support the system, such as potassium chloride or calcium and sodium phosphate. If your child has had antibiotics, the immune system needs to be built up with vitamins A, C and E. The supplements acidophilus and bifidus may also be recommended.

Osteopathy Osteopaths believe that if there is some sort of restriction in the cranial or spinal area, perhaps due to a long-forgotten fall or accident, then there can be an imbalance of pressure between the outer and middle ear, leading to a build-up of fluid. This can affect the tension in the eardrum and result in a loss of hearing – a sign of glue ear. Work will involve releasing tension in the relevant areas of the cranium or spine.

Acupuncture Western medicine tends to treat glue ear by draining the fluid and may involve an operation to insert grommets to help this process. Acupuncture will try to treat the cause to stop the build-up of fluid occurring in the first place. An acupuncturist will see the problem as an imbalance of heat, damp and congestion. The condition may worsen for the first four or five treatments, as it is designed to break up the phlegm in the head and body and get it to 'move out'. As well as acupuncture, the practitioner may advise avoiding dairy products, as these can exacerbate the damp, spicy foods, as these create heat, and flour as this helps to promote congestion.

Other therapies that may be beneficial: reflexology, aromatherapy, chiropractic.

'We first became concerned about James when we were told he was trailing behind at school. His teacher said he wasn't paying attention as much as he should, but she thought it seemed to be more a case of him not being able to hear rather than deliberately not listening. He'd always had problems with his ears.

Whenever he got a cold he always got an ear infection, too, and he just seemed to finish one course of antibiotics before he'd be starting another.

'The doctor said he had glue ear – a build-up of fluid in the ear. He had a hearing aid fitted and was on the waiting list to have an operation for grommets to be inserted which would help the fluid to drain away.

'I can't remember who suggested trying osteopathy, but we thought we'd give it a go if there was a chance James might not need an operation. The osteopath examined him and said he had found strain patterns often due to a traumatic birth and asked whether James had had a difficult delivery. I was amazed that something as long ago as his birth could be affecting him, but, in fact, it had been a traumatic labour which had lasted for hours ending up with James so distressed, he had to be delivered by emergency Caesarian. Over a number of sessions, these strains were addressed and James's hearing returned to normal. He no longer has a hearing aid and didn't need the op.'

Danny and James, 8

HAYFEVER (allergic rhinitis)

Allergic rhinitis, commonly known as hayfever, can occur at any time of year, depending on what your child is allergic to. In the spring, allergy to tree pollens will trigger it off, in the summer, various grasses, and in autumn, with the damp weather, moulds can cause problems. The sufferer reacts against these triggers, known as allergens. For some reason, the immune system over-reacts and releases antibodies and histamine, which lead to symptoms such as a runny nose, watery eyes, sneezing and congestion. The child may also feel more tired and irritable as they cope with the symptoms of the allergy. Children with hayfever may also suffer from related diseases such as asthma or eczema. They are also more likely to suffer if any of these conditions run in the family.

What you can do

Try to minimize contact with known allergens. Take note of the day's pollen count during the summer and keep doors and windows, including car windows, closed during high count days. Regularly clean your child's mattress, bed covers and any soft furnishings that pollen can cling to. An ionizer may help to filter the air. Get your children some fun sunglasses – they'll love them and they will also keep airborne particles from entering the eyes (although be sure they have a proper ultra-violet filter to prevent eye damage).

Treatment

Naturopathy A naturopath would aim to build up the immune system and general health of the child to help the body fight off what it sees as foreign invaders. To help this, dairy products, which help to produce mucus, may need to be eliminated from the diet. Fresh fruit and vegetables in the diet would be emphasized and vitamin and mineral salt supplements may be advised.

Acupuncture Practitioners find acupuncture can work well in treating hayfever, eczema and asthma, although it does depend on the individual child. It stimulates the points relating to the large intestine, spleen and lungs, relieving symptoms and related stress.

Herbal medicine Plantain, which acts as an expectorant, may be advised. Elderflower also contains properties which will help ease catarrhal inflammation, and Nettles, which act as an astringent and tonic, may prove beneficial.

Reflexology To help combat hayfever, the part of the foot worked on will relate to the adrenal glands which produce adrenaline, the 'fight or flight' hormone and can help stop the body from over-reacting to supposed invaders or allergens. The endocrine system will also be worked on as the endocrine glands help to regulate the internal functions of the body.

Biochemic tissue salts A homoeopath, naturopath or herbalist may also give your child tissue salts. These may be given individually for particular symptoms such as runny nose and watery eyes or for the mucus, or they may be given Combination H, which contains more than one tissue salt which may be able to help relieve symptoms.

Other therapies that may be beneficial: homoeopathy, hypnotherapy, osteopathy.

'I suffer from hayfever, so when my daughter started getting similar symptoms – sneezing, coughing and runny nose – I knew she probably had it too. I decided to try a naturopath because I knew that their philosophy of the body treating itself could help in preventing Julia from developing other allergies and asthma, which I also get.

'The first visit took over an hour. The naturopath checked Julia's eyes, tongue and nails as part of her diagnosis. Just from looking at her eyes she said Julia seemed to have bowel problems. She was right – Julia has had watery stools since she was born. We went through my diet when breastfeeding, Julia's diet since starting solids and what conventional treatment, such as antibiotics, she'd ever had, to build up a complete picture of her health.

'We were advised to take Julia completely off dairy products for a while as her system was overloaded which was helping to produce the excess mucus she'd been suffering as part of the hayfever.

'I was a bit apprehensive about how we'd manage, but Julia

didn't even notice swapping to goats' milk and we just have to make sure she gets her calcium from other sources. Although she is still mucusy, it has helped.'

Pauline and Julia, 13 months

HEADACHE

Children often complain of headaches, but there is rarely a serious cause. It may be due to a related problem, such as ear ache or sinusitis (see under relevant alphabetical section) or may be due to anxiety over something, over-tiredness or over-exertion.

What you can do

Watch out for other symptoms such as ear ache or raised temperature. The child may be overheated, so open a window or go for a walk, or if they prefer, lie them down in a darkened room. Check your child has not had a fall or been injured, which may be causing the headache. Try to get them to relax as much as possible. One study found that relaxation training helped to increase headache-free days by 15 per cent.

Treatment

Naturopathy The practitioner will try to find a link to the headaches. The cause may be dehydration. A naturopath will ask about the child's frequency of urinating, bowel habits and how many times they drink during the day. Their diet will be looked at in case a food intolerance, for example to cheese or chocolate, may be a trigger. Mineral and vitamins may be deficient so mineral salts such as magnesium and potassium phosphates and an increase in vitamins B and C may be recommended. Cooling or warming compresses may be applied to soothe any neck or head tensions, as well as massage, which can be taught to the parent. Herbal medicine may also be used to strengthen the nervous system and give pain relief.

Chiropractic The chiropractor would first rule out any serious causes of recurrent headaches before examining for neck joint and muscular dysfunction. If the chiropractor finds a structural problem, they will use appropriate manipulation and mobilization of the affected joints, according to the child's age. If this isn't able to correct the problem, other possible imbalances will be checked for, for instance in the jaw or pelvis, which may be exacerbating the condition. Advice will also be given on posture and ergonomics.

Osteopathy An osteopath may see the headache as being caused by a mechanical imbalance in the body, with tension leading to increased muscle tone in the neck and head. Suppression in the cranial area may interfere with the function of the arteries and veins, leading to congestion and inflammation, so an osteopath would work on this area to bring relief.

Aromatherapy If your child suffers from headaches or migraine, an aromatherapist may use a combination of oils to help bring relief. Roman Chamomile has properties which act as an analgesic as well as helping to soothe the nerves. Lemon may also be used as it helps to stimulate the body to produce white corpuscles to help fight off infection, of which a headache may be just one symptom.

Caution

If symptoms include temperature, a stiff neck, lethargy and a dislike of bright lights, it may be a sign of a more dangerous condition, such as meningitis (see *Meningitis*) or encephalitis, and medical help should be immediately called.

Other therapies that may be beneficial: biochemic tissue salts, acupuncture.

'My daughter is a violinist and, like most successful musicians, started to learn when she was very young. But when she reached her teens she began suffering terrible headaches whenever she played. She also said her left knee was quite often painful. Both her foot arches had dropped as well which meant that it became difficult for her to walk after about ten minutes.

'We took her to the GP who referred her on to a physiotherapist. She had many weeks of sessions, but her headaches, aches and pains continued. It was becoming more and more difficult to motivate herself to play, so we decided to try something else. Someone suggested the McTimoney form of chiropractic, as it is very gentle and works on the whole body, not just the area in pain, as we thought all her problems may be linked.

'After six sessions all her symptoms were gone and she was back to her normal self and relieved that she could play without pain. That was three years ago and she's had no problems since.'

Patrick and Elisabeth, now 16

INFLUENZA ('flu)

Influenza, or 'flu, has similar but more severe symptoms than the common cold, such as a raised temperature, chills, headaches, sweating, aching and tired muscles, sore throat and a loss of appetite. And, as with the cold, 'flu can easily be passed on in classrooms by coughing and sneezing and can occur in epidemics. The symptoms usually only last a few days but can be up to a week. As the immune system is weakened, other infections may set in such as bronchitis, sinusitis or ear ache (see under relevant alphabetical sections). It may also make other conditions, such as asthma, worse.

What you can do

Keep your child warm and comfortable in a well-ventilated room. Make sure they drink plenty of fluids and if uninterested in eating, try some 'easy' foods such as soup or a boiled egg and toasted soldiers. Monitor their temperature and watch for signs of any secondary infection developing.

Treatment

Naturopathy Naturopaths work towards preventing illnesses such as 'flu through a healthy diet and lifestyle. Recommendations may include Elderflower tea to help the fever, eating vitamin C-rich foods such as citrus fruits and strawberries to boost the immune system, and zinc, needed to help fight infection and found in vegetables, and garlic, for its antiviral properties. Your child should rest until their temperature returns to normal. The fever should not be suppressed as it's the body's way of fighting infection. The naturopath may also recommend a pack placed around the child's trunk, where a cold water sheet is wrung out and wrapped around the body and then covered with warm blankets. Plenty of water will also be useful, preferably added to homemade juices. Fruit may also be given to help detoxify the body, and mineral salts such as potassium chloride and iron phosphate to help the body fight infection.

Biochemic tissue salts To help reduce fever and suppress a cough, Ferr. phos. may help, or Kali. sulph. to promote sweating out the illness. Once your child is beginning to recover, but is still feeling weak with no appetite after their illness, use Combination B. Combination Q will help act as a decongestant.

Traditional Chinese medicine Chinese medicine believes that 'flu falls into three categories – wind heat, wind cold and damp, and treatment will be according to one of these diagnoses. Plenty of fluids to flush out the body's toxins will be advised. Moxibustion, where heated needles or moxa sticks are held over the acupuncture points on the body to release any blockages to the flow of Qi or vital energy, may also be applied. A practitioner may prescribe a mixture of Dandelion, Marigold, Garlic, Cardamom and Chrysanthemum, among others, to help relieve symptoms.

Reflexology Children can be very susceptible to infections. A reflexologist would work on the areas corresponding to the site of infection, such as a sore throat, but will also pay particular attention to the area of the foot relating to the adrenal glands, as it is these glands which help to activate the responses to fight off infection.

Other therapies that may be beneficial: homoeopathy, Bach Flower Remedies.

LARYNGITIS

Laryngitis is usually caused by a viral or bacterial infection, such as a cold, which leads to the inflammation of the larynx or voice box. The child will become hoarse and may completely lose their voice. It may hurt to swallow and may be accompanied by a dry cough, raised temperature and sore throat.

What you can do

Keep your child quiet and try to prevent them from talking. Keep an eye on their temperature and look for signs of secondary infection, such as bronchitis. Warm drinks with honey will soothe their sore throats. It will help the cough if the room is kept humidified. This can be done by placing bowls of water near hot radiators, or humidifiers can be bought in department stores.

Treatment

Aromatherapy Steam inhalations using Chamomile, Lavender and Thyme may be prescribed by the therapist to help to soothe the throat. Massaging the neck area may also be recommended with oils such as Chamomile, Lemon, Thyme or Geranium.

Bach Flower Remedies Your child's personality is the key to selecting the correct Bach Flower Remedy. Children who feel sorry for themselves and grumble about how ill they feel would be given Willow, while those who are too impatient to wait for their throats to recover and get up and start shouting too soon would be helped with Impatiens. Crab Apple is also useful as a cleansing remedy and Olive will help deal with the physical tiredness resulting from the illness.

Herbal medicine There are a variety of herbs that a practitioner may recommend for the inflammation. Red or Garden Sage or Lady's Mantle may be given in a dose to gargle with, and particularly Balm of Gilead if your child has lost their voice. Propolis spray or lozenges also work well.

Naturopathy A naturopath will look at possible causes for the laryngitis. It could be poor elimination, particularly if the child has a diet high in refined foods such as white sugar and flour or eats a lot of sweets. Or if the problem is recurrent, it may be a sign of a food allergy, for instance to dairy products or wheat. Epsom salt baths to help detoxify the body may be recommended or a short course diet of three days on just fruit, under supervision, may be advised. Gargling with a weak solution of salt (ensure none is swallowed), lemon and a drop of Myrrh or Golden Seal may help. Mineral salt supplements and an increase in vitamins C, A, E and zinc may be recommended. It may also help to wrap the throat in cotton cloth soaked in tepid water which should be left on for an hour at a time, as this will help to stimulate healing by increasing the circulation and lymph flow to the area.

Caution

Consult your doctor if symptoms persist for more than five

days, as a secondary infection, such as croup, bronchitis or tonsillitis, may have set in.

Other therapies that may be beneficial: reflexology, traditional Chinese medicine, homoeopathy, osteopathy.

LICE

Once one child at school has head lice, others soon follow as they can be easily passed on by direct contact such as a child scratching her head and touching another child, not necessarily on their head. Lice are not fussy and are just as happy on a clean head of hair as on a dirty one, so your child's hygiene is irrelevant. The lice live by sucking blood from the scalp. The bite marks will itch intensely and scratching can lead to infection or inflammation. The proliferate lice lay tiny pale eggs (nits) which stick firmly to the hair and look like dandruff, except are difficult to remove. Once the eggs have hatched, the new batch of lice will live off the scalp and survive for several weeks.

What you can do

Once you've discovered your child has lice, inform their school or nursery and playmates. Check the rest of the family for infestation. Strong-smelling shampoos and lotions can be bought from the chemist to get rid of the lice. However, these often have side-effects due to the strong chemicals used, which can be toxic and provoke allergic reactions. Tea-Tree shampoo is a natural alternative, although you will need several washes for it to be effective. The dead lice and nits should then be removed with a fine-tooth comb.

Treatment

Aromatherapy To avoid the use of strong chemical shampoos to zap the lice and nits, an aromatherapist may make up a shampoo containing Rosemary, Eucalyptus and Sweet

Thyme. A hair rinse and scalp tonic may also be given to prevent further infestations.

Herbal medicine Herbalists may recommend Sassafras which works well on skin problems and acts as a disinfectant. Aniseed works as a parasiticide and the use of its oil can help control lice. The bitter effects of Quassia, if given in lotion form, may also be useful.

MEASLES

Measles is a common and highly contagious viral disease. It is spread by airborne nasal secretions. Symptoms include runny nose, sore eyes, dry cough, raised temperature, headaches, small white spots in the mouth and, after a few days, a brown-red rash will start to cover the upper body. The lymph glands may also become enlarged. It may take an incubation period of eight to ten days for these symptoms to appear and the child will then be contagious from the start of this time to a week after the onset. Lesser complications such as chest or ear infections may develop. In children under five, there is also the slight possibility of febrile convulsions, when the child loses consciousness and the limbs twitch uncontrollably for a short time. More serious complications include encephalitis or inflammation of the brain.

The MMR (measles/mumps/rubella) vaccine is routinely given to children aged about fifteen months. Although the number of cases of measles has been reduced, many children who now catch measles have already had the vaccine (see *Vaccination*).

What you can do

Once diagnosis has been confirmed, make sure the child drinks plenty of fluids. Try to keep their temperature down by sponging with tepid water. Their eyes may also be sore and bathing them in warm water or eye drops may help. Look out for complications such as ear ache.

Treatment

Medical diagnosis should be sought, but the following therapies may be beneficial:

Homoeopathy Although little can be done about the appearance of spots, the other symptoms may be helped. Gelsemium may be prescribed by a homoeopath to help reduce the raised temperature and headache, as well as possible associations such as thirst and constipation. Euphrasia will help the runny nose and sore eyes. If the child is feeling very restless and irritable due to their illness, Pulsatilla may work as well as helping to clear the cough and catarrh from the nose and throat.

Herbal medicine A herbalist may recommend a general increase in vitamin C to help fight off infection. A mixture of herbs, such as Golden Seal to help reduce runny nose and sore eyes, Chamomile to calm the child, Echinacea to deal with the infection, and Marigold if the glands are swollen, may be prescribed.

Traditional Chinese medicine A practitioner may advise infusions or decoctions to help reduce what they see as heat in the blood and stomach. These may include Safflower, Peppermint, Marigold and Yarrow. A cooling solution of Lavender may be applied to the spots.

Naturopathy A naturopath will recommend boosting the immune system to help fight off infection, so an increase in foods containing vitamins A, C and E and also zinc, which can be found in fruit and vegetables, will be recommended. Mineral salt supplements, such as iron, magnesium and potassium phosphates and potassium chloride may also be given. However, at first your child will probably not want to eat much food, although drinking water should be encouraged. Foods that encourage the production of mucus should be cut back, such as dairy products. If the child is suffering from itching, a tepid bath containing oatmeal should help bring relief. Herbal remedies, such as Yarrow, Chamomile, Skull-cap, Cleavers and Golden Seal may also be given.

Caution

If your child's temperature is over 40°C (104°F), their breathing is shallow, they have chest pain or lose conscious-ness, seek medical help immediately.

Other therapies that may be beneficial: reflexology, aromather-apy, Bach Flower Remedies, biochemic tissue salts.

MENINGITIS

Meningitis is the inflammation of the meninges or mem-branes which cover the brain and spinal cord. There are two types. Viral meningitis is the milder form, and tends to occur after mumps, with symptoms similar to 'flu. It does not usually need treatment, although pain relief may be necessary. Bacterial meningitis, and its most common form, meningo-coccal meningitis, is very serious and if you suspect your child has it, seek immediate medical attention, as it can be fatal. Symptoms include a raised temperature, stiff neck, headache, nausea, vomiting and sometimes a dislike of light and lethargy. In children under eighteen months the fontanelle may bulge. Symptoms can develop in just a few hours and there may also be a red rash. Your child may need a lumbar puncture to remove fluid from the spinal cord for definite diagnosis. Massive amounts of intravenous antibiotics will be given if your child is suffering from meningitis to try and kill off the bacteria.

What you can do

If your child has been diagnosed with meningitis, doctors will do their best to halt the infection. Although there is little you can physically do to help your child once they are in hospital, knowing you are close will help. Inform any friends and your child's school so that parents may be on the lookout for symptoms.

Treatment

Medical attention should be sought immediately, but the following complementary therapies may also be beneficial in aftercare:

Osteopathy An osteopath will try to help boost the immune system after the effects of the disease and subsequent doses of antibiotics. This may include working through the cranial system so that the efficiency of the lymphatic system, which is an important part of the immune system and helps to fight off infection, can be improved. The meninges will also be treated for scar tissue and the effects of the inflammation.

Herbal medicine There are herbs which can help the body to protect itself against infection and reinforce the work of the antibiotics. Echinacea, Wild Indigo and St John's Wort all have antibacterial and antiviral properties and may be given in an infusion.

Homoeopathy Any homoeopathic remedies advised after an attack of meningitis will be given to help the child's constitution and to build up the immune system depleted after a severe illness.

Naturopathy Following the use of antibiotics given to treat meningitis, the immune system will be depleted and need rebuilding. Probiotics (which counter the effects of antibiotics), such as acidophilus and bifidus, will be recommended as well as increased intakes of vitamin C, the B vitamins, which will help to support the nervous system, and herbs such as Echinacea, Cinnamon and Cleavers. Mineral salt supplements, which help to support the body's functions, such as potassium, magnesium and calcium phosphates and potassium chloride may be given. The child's overall diet should be rich in nutrients, using organic food rather than processed. Other treatment will be given, depending on what damage has occurred to the nervous system and any secondary infections. Plenty of rest, gentle exercise and fresh air will all help on the road to recovery.

Other therapies that may be beneficial in aftercare, for instance in helping to boost the immune system: aromatherapy, traditional Chinese medicine.

MIGRAINE

Migraine is a severe headache, which in children is usually accompanied by abdominal pain. Some sufferers also experience flashing lights and numbness on the affected part of the head. Migraine is prone to run in families and can affect children as young as three. Although some children get a one-off, they do tend to recur. It can be triggered by any number of things from a change in routine to excitement, worry or an adverse reaction to food. Common food culprits are dairy products, chocolate, red meat (particularly pork), caffeine, yeast products and acidic foods. A migraine may last from a couple of hours to a day or more. Children particularly tend to recover once they have vomited. Painkillers will bring relief. If your child suffers more frequent attacks, drugs may be prescribed to give at the onset.

What you can do

If the migraines occur less than once a month, treatment for that attack as it happens is probably all that is needed. Monitor what triggers your child's attack, so that you can try to prevent future ones. Keep them in a cool, darkened room and leave a bucket next to the bed in case they are sick.

Treatment

Herbal medicine If your child suffers from recurrent migraines, a herbalist will be able to make up a preparation to take at the onset of an attack, to reduce symptoms. This may include Chamomile, Oats, Skullcap, Vervain, Hops, Hyssop and Wood Betony.

Chiropractic A chiropractor will first check to see whether the migraines are linked to trigger factors, such as an allergy to a certain food. If not, there may be a skeletal cause, originating from a birth trauma or a fall. The child will be examined for structural imbalances in the pelvis, lower back and, most importantly, in the neck and jaw. Any problems found will be treated with the appropriate manipulation and mobilizing techniques to help correct them.

Acupressure To help alleviate symptoms, hold the child's hand and press from the end of the crease between the thumb and first finger towards the first finger bone.

Reflexology The big toe relates to the head in reflexology so the therapist would concentrate on this area. The areas relating to the spine and neck would also be worked on to help release tension. The whole foot would also be manipulated to treat the body as a whole.

Other therapies that may be beneficial: aromatherapy, Alexander Technique, osteopathy.

'I took my daughter Florence to a reflexologist because she was only seven but suffered from terrible migraines. I'd take her after school with her two sisters and brother and they'd sit watching cartoons while the reflexologist went to work.

'Alison worked on the whole foot, but said she was also paying particular attention to the lymphatic system to help fight infection. She also worked on the large and small intestines as when

Florence had an attack it always started off by her being sick. Sometimes she'd been in bed for three days at a time with it.

'We went every week for a few months and the period of time between attacks became longer and she recovered more quickly after an attack, too. We stopped going with the arrival of the summer holidays, but if things get bad again, I'll take her back.'

Deborah and Florence, 7

MUMPS

Mumps is a viral illness that causes the salivary glands to swell on either one or both sides of the jaw. It used to be very common until the introduction of the MMR (mumps/measles/rubella) vaccine. There is an incubation period of fourteen to twenty-one days and the child may be infectious for a week before and up to two weeks after the appearance of symptoms. Your child may seem unwell for a couple of days before the symptoms appear, when the glands will then begin to swell. They may find it difficult to swallow as the mouth dries up and have a raised temperature and headache. Painkillers may be given. In older children, the testes may be painful in boys, while girls may experience lower abdominal pain.

What you can do

Your child will be finding it difficult to swallow, due to the lack of saliva, so liquidize food so it will slip down easily. Soups, yoghurt and milkshakes are all easy for them to sip. Make sure they drink plenty of fluids.

Treatment

Medical diagnosis should be sought, but the following therapies may be beneficial:

Homoeopathy When the symptoms are first noticed, a

homoeopath may recommend Aconite to help relieve the pain, thirst and fever. Belladonna may also be prescribed if the right side of the face is affected and Rhus. tox. if the left side is swollen. The latter may also help to prevent symptoms occurring if your child has come into contact with a child already affected.

Herbal medicine An infusion of Cleavers and St John's Wort, which have anti-inflammatory properties, may prove beneficial and Echinacea may also be recommended by a herbalist to stimulate the immune system.

Osteopathy To help boost the immune system after a case of mumps, an osteopath may work on the cranial system to alleviate mechanical strains in the body. This can improve the flow and interchange of the body's fluids, such as lymph (which plays an important part in the immune system) and blood.

Reflexology A reflexologist would work on the base of the big toe that relates to the throat and neck area and the areas that relate to the head in general. Treatment would also include working on the lymphatic system to help fight off infection.

Caution

If symptoms persist for more than ten days, consult your doctor, as there may be complications such as meningitis.

Other therapies that may be beneficial: naturopathy, reflexology, traditional Chinese medicine.

'John had a mild case of mumps, but he was still feeling pretty poorly. I was told there wasn't much we could do except wait it out and keep him well rested and quiet. I wanted to do something positive for him, so I asked a reflexologist friend of mine to come and see him.

'He loved all the attention and was quite happy to lie there while she 'played' with his feet and we all chatted about his condition. I don't know what part of the foot represents what, except that the toes represent the head area and the big toe in particular was worked on. But she covered the whole foot as his whole body was obviously suffering from the effects of the infection through fatigue and just generally feeling rotten.

'By the next day, although he was still suffering, he said he felt a lot less uncomfortable and I'm sure it helped him to get better a lot more quickly than if he'd had nothing done to help him.'

Shirley and John, 12

NAPPY RASH

Most babies get nappy rash at some time. Symptoms include inflamed skin, small red spots and the smell of ammonia. It occurs when a nappy has been left on too long, so that the urine and faeces begin to break down, releasing ammonia which irritates the skin. If you use towelling nappies, it may also be caused by an allergic reaction to your washing powder or fabric conditioner and could be a sign that your child has eczema.

What you can do

Keep your baby's nappy off for as long as you dare, so that air can freely circulate. Change nappies regularly, every two to three hours and after every motion, and cleanse the whole area thoroughly but gently, before patting dry. Use a mild emollient to help protect the skin, particularly at night.

Treatment

Aromatherapy For persistent nappy rash, a practitioner may recommend a massage oil to gently rub into the affected area. Frankincense might be used for its regenerative and antiseptic qualities, Lavender to soothe inflamed skin and Geranium to help cleanse. Add three drops of one of these oils to a dessertspoon (10ml) of a carrier oil such as Sweet Almond and warm the hands before applying. Or gently wash the rash with cotton wool dipped in a pint of warm water to which a drop each of Yarrow and Lavender or Chamomile German and Lavender have been well mixed.

Herbal medicine Prevention, by regularly changing your baby's nappy, is the best cure. But even the most regularly cleaned backsides can get the odd rash. Creams or ointments containing Calendula, which acts as an anti-inflammatory, will help soothe the skin. If the rash is persistent, a practitioner may recommend compresses containing Chamomile or Marigold, both of which will help to calm the skin down. Buchu and Cleavers may also be prescribed to help reduce the acidity of the urine.

Homoeopathy If the homoeopath finds the baby's urine is particularly acidic, Merc. sol. may be recommended. If the skin is very raw red, Cantharis may be used and Rhus tox. if the skin has come up in sore, raised spots. For home use, ointments containing Calendula and Marigold will help to soothe the skin.

Diet If you are breastfeeding, restrict eating spicy foods and alcohol and any foods that you are aware of that may irritate your baby's digestive system.

Caution

Check your baby's mouth for small white spots which may indicate thrush, as this can contribute to nappy rash, in which case treatment for fungal infection should be included.

NIGHTMARES/NIGHT TERRORS

Most children will suffer nightmares at some point, particularly those aged between eight and ten. They are unpleasant dreams which occur during REM (rapid eye movement) sleep. The child may partially or fully awake and be crying and panicky and will probably be able to recall the dream. They are more likely to occur when the child's breathing is hindered in some way, for example if they are suffering from a cold or illness.

Night terrors also commonly occur in children, but happen during NREM (non-rapid eye movement) sleep, and usually start in children aged between four and seven. On suddenly waking in fear and screaming, the child will feel frightened and may not be sure who you are or where they are. They will have no memory of the event the next morning. The odd dream or terror is normal in children, but if they are happening on a frequent and regular basis, there may be an underlying problem which needs to be addressed.

What you can do

Comfort your child as soon as possible and let them know you are close. Cuddle and soothe them until they calm down, but don't try to make them remember what their dream or terror was about. If their sleep is being frequently disturbed by these night wakings, choose a time during the day to try and discuss any anxieties or problems with your child to see if they are the root cause.

Treatment

Hypnotherapy A hypnotherapist will use the unconscious mind to learn things that can be useful and to rid the child of nightmares or night terrors. This may include resourcing the child's memory to look at the past when nightmares did not affect them and to disassociate night time as a time of possible fear. The child will then be taught to use those resources to cope with any fears they have in the present.

Bach Flower Remedies There are various remedies that can help your child. Rock Rose will help ease the child's panic on waking and calm the fright from the dream. If the child is hysterical and out of control, Cherry Plum will help to soothe them. Rescue Remedy contains both these remedies and so will be helpful. If the child is fearful, for instance worrying that a parent is going to leave home, Mimulus may help, while Honeysuckle may help a child who suffers a recurrent nightmare because they are reliving a bad experience.

Traditional Chinese medicine The Chinese see fright and heat as the most common cause of nightmares. In children under three, slow bowel movement and the stagnation of food may also be seen as a cause. A cooling evening drink such as Chrysanthemum Flower may be given and a variety of herbs may be prescribed. Acupuncture can also achieve very quick results in two or three treatments.

'My wife and I were becoming completely exhausted because our youngest child, Natalie, was suffering from nightmares and was terrified of the dark. We don't know what triggered it off, but it was obviously something deep inside her that had changed her from a happy to a sombre little girl. She began waking up screaming. It wasn't always easy to understand what she was afraid of, but it seemed to be about giant animals with scaly backs coming to get her in the dark. She goes to sleep quite happily, but then she wakes up, terrified. It had got to a point where we'd both be lying in bed, just waiting for her cry.

'First of all we tried counselling to get to the bottom of it. Then psychotherapy, neither of which helped. She was even put on medication, which we weren't too happy about as she's so young, but we didn't know what else to do. Then a family friend suggested hypnosis. We were a little doubtful, but she was getting worse and nothing else had worked.

'I didn't go to the sessions myself, but I understand she was taken back to times when she was happy and not scared of any giant animals. After the first session the nightmares disappeared and by the third, she was back to her old self.'

Jeremy and Natalie, 6

NOSEBLEED

Nosebleeds are common in children as they tend to start after a knock to the nose or by hard blowing, causing the mucous membranes inside the nose to rupture and leak blood. It can be alarming if there is a lot of blood, but unless the nosebleed persists for more than twenty minutes, they are not usually serious.

What you can do

Don't try to staunch the blood flow by putting anything up the child's nose. Lean their head forwards over the sink or towel and make sure the mouth is slightly open so they can breathe normally. Tell them not to sniff or blow as this could start the bleeding again. They should also avoid leaning backwards, as blood will drip down the back of the nose and throat and may cause vomiting.

Treatment

Naturopathy A naturopath will assess the child's overall stress levels, as this can often lead to nose-picking. Otherwise, dry conditions such as central heating, over-blowing the nose or cold sores can all be causes. If the child has low zinc levels and too little bioflavonoids and vitamin C in the diet, this can affect the blood capillaries which become more fragile and will be slow to heal if burst. An increase in foods rich in vitamins A, C, E, and in zinc, garlic, water, fruit and vegetables may be recommended. Also mineral salt supplements such as sodium and potassium phosphates may be given.

Herbal medicine A herbalist may recommend Oil of Cypress dropped on to cotton wool and gently sniffed to help to reduce the nosebleed more quickly. Other herbs that may help and are known for their astringent qualities are Witch Hazel, Yarrow and St John's Wort. To toughen up the mucous membranes, a tincture of Golden Seal, which acts as a useful astringent, given three times a day for children over two years old, may help. For children under two, Yarrow, which also has astringent as well as antiseptic qualities, may be advised instead.

Homoeopathy If your child is prone to nosebleeds, usually because the child picks at their nose, a homoeopath may recommend Ferrum phos. If the child is agitated and anxious, Arsenicum to help calm them may also be advised.

Bach Flower Remedies A practitioner may recommend that children who repeatedly cause nosebleeds by always blowing their noses too hard or picking them may be helped by Chestnut Bud. Rescue Remedy is good for the shock and fear caused by a bad nosebleed and any squeamishness at the sight of blood may be helped by giving Crab Apple.

Caution

If the nosebleed continues for longer than twenty minutes or started after a hard knock to your child's head, consult a doctor immediately as an X-ray may be needed in case of a skull fracture, or the rupture may need to be cauterized – sealed with heat. Also consult a doctor if there is a recurrent nosebleed to exclude any abnormality in the clotting process.

Other therapies that may be beneficial: osteopathy, traditional Chinese medicine, chiropractic.

'Sanjay was taken to a medical herbalist because he'd been suffering from nosebleeds for five years. Every morning and evening as he bent over the bathroom sink to brush his teeth, his nose would pour blood. The herbalist checked that he was otherwise healthy and that there wasn't a more serious underlying problem causing the bleeding. But he'd had numerous tests and his blood pressure was fine. He was healthy in every other way and had a good, traditional Indian diet – lentils, chapatis and so on.

'The herbalist looked up his nose and said that it was very inflamed and irritated. She gave Sanjay a tincture to drink which contained Golden Seal and Bay Berry, saying that both acted as astringents and the Golden Seal in particular would help the mucous-membrane lining. And to help the damaged tissue she gave herbs of Marigold and Horsetail.

'He had enough herbs for four weeks, but after a week, the nosebleeds had stopped so he didn't need to take them anymore.'

Renu and Sanjay, now 15

PHOBIAS (and fears)

Phobia is the irrational fear of a particular object or situation and many start in childhood. The most common of these can start at a young age and are known as simple phobias, for instance fear of an animal such as dogs, cats or spiders. Often the animal in question can be largely avoided, but for some children it can become a big problem. Older children can suffer from fears like being fearful of situations such as eating in public or having to write in front of others. Agoraphobia can also affect later teenage years, when the child becomes fearful of open places. When confronted with the source of their phobia or anxiety, the child may become extremely anxious and panicky. It is thought that simple phobias, such as the fear of spiders, may be passed on by family conditioning – if the mother is afraid of spiders, the child too will become fearful. Or the child may have been badly scared by a spider when small and has not overcome the incident. There are also some theories that phobias are a symbol of some deeper problem.

Behavioural therapy is commonly used in treating fears and phobias. This may involve slowly increasing exposure to the cause of the phobia. Relaxation techniques will also be used to help reduce stress. Alternatively, flooding may be used, when the patient, supported by their therapist, is fully exposed to the source of their anxiety.

What you can do

The fear or phobia may be manageable by avoiding its cause. If your child is afraid of an animal or insect, try to minimize any exposure. This can obviously prove difficult and, if the child's fear is causing problems in normal family life, some sort of therapy may be needed to overcome it.

Treatment

Hypnotherapy Hypnotherapists will use techniques to help the child use their unconscious mind to learn and rid them of their phobia. For instance, a child who is scared of anything coloured red will not need to be regressed back to when they were hit by a red car to get rid of their phobia, but will learn to disassociate the colour red with a negative feeling. Instead, positive feelings about the colour red may be suggested.

Kinesiology A practitioner will use different balancing methods and muscle testing to help dispel any phobias or fears that the child is experiencing. The stomach would be particularly worked on, as it is seen as the organ related to both rational and irrational emotional stress. Phobias can obviously cause a lot of stress, so this will be worked on as mental stress can affect the body in other ways.

Acupuncture The Chinese say that 'at seven, children fall from heaven'. This means that they develop their own emotions, rebelliousness and possibly phobias. Until that age any phobia is more likely to be a mirror of a parental phobia, such as a fear of spiders. Treatment will usually be directed at giving the child self-confidence and self-awareness, and strengthening the kidney meridian which is held to be linked with fears and anxiety.

Bach Flower Remedies The Remedies treat the emotions rather than the illness, so are useful in helping children's fears and may help to generate positive feelings. There are different remedies that can be given depending on the type of fear – Mimulus may be given for known worries, while Aspen may be given for unknown fears which leads them to being generally anxious, and Rock Rose for panic and terror.

Other therapies that may be beneficial: aromatherapy, reflexology, acupressure, homoeopathy, herbal medicine, massage.

'Mark is a very fearful child. He's afraid of the firebell at his school. I don't know why as he's never been able to explain it, but the sound of it makes him very nervous and anxious. He gets frightened about other things too, and a lot of the time he can't say why. But then sometimes he's very articulate. He's a very timid child who doesn't have a lot of confidence and finds it difficult to mix with other children. This makes him very clingy. I tried Bach Flower Remedies and gave him Mimulus which helps treat the fear of known things to combat his worries about the firebell. I also gave him Larch to help build up his confidence. He took these for two weeks and other remedies were added and taken away, depending on how he was doing. So I gave him Aspen for a while which helps deal with unknown fears, and Chicory to help with the clinginess. Now he's really improved and has a lot

more confidence. I used to have to walk him right into the class-
room before he'd let go of my hand, but now I can just take him
to the corner of the road and he's quite happy to go into school
all by himself.'

Julie and Mark, 8

RASH (Heat)

Heat rash, also known as prickly heat, is particularly common
in babies as their sweat glands are not yet sophisticated
enough to regulate temperature. It occurs when the body
becomes overheated and sweat is unable to evaporate, blocking the glands. Symptoms include small, itchy red spots
spreading across the neck, face, shoulders, chest and in the
creases of elbows, knees, armpits and nappy area. Once the
child has cooled down, the rash should eventually disappear.

What you can do

Cool your baby in a tepid (not cold) bath or sponge down the
skin. Dry them thoroughly, particularly in the folds of the
skin. Make sure there is a circulation of air in the room and
any heating is turned down. Put on only light cotton clothing.

Treatment

Aromatherapy An aromatherapist may recommend a bath
containing two drops of Roman Chamomile, a useful anti-
inflammatory, one drop of Lavender, soothing for inflamed
skin, and one drop of Sandalwood, for relaxing, which should
help to calm the skin. For babies under a year, mixing
together ¼ cup of baking soda and two drops of Lavender,
before adding to a tepid bath, has been effective.

Herbal medicine Calendula ointment or lotion can help to
soothe the rash, particularly if also mixed with a little Aloe
Vera gel. Or a poultice of nettles soaked in a bowl of warm

water and applied to the skin may be recommended. A cold compress using a couple of drops of Lavender, or a cold infusion of Marigold may also be beneficial.

Homoeopathy A homoeopath will look at how the child is reacting to the rash as well as discussing the symptoms and will give a remedy accordingly. For instance, if the child is also hot and feverish, Belladonna may be given.

Acupuncture An acupuncturist would choose the energy points in the body that may help to eliminate the toxins causing the rash, dispersing it and re-balancing the body. Using points to boost the immune system will help to prevent further outbreaks.

Caution

If the symptoms have not disappeared after twelve hours consult a doctor in case there is another cause for the rash.

'My son started getting rashes over his body when he was about two months old – just after he'd had his first set of vaccinations. I took him to the doctor who said he probably had eczema and wanted to give Joe cortisone cream. I didn't think it was eczema, but more probably some sort of heat rash and wasn't happy about giving him the cream. I've used various alternative therapies in the past and I knew that the rash was a sign of something trying to come out and that it shouldn't be suppressed.

'I decided to try acupuncture. I can see why some parents might be daunted by having needles stuck into their children, but Joe really didn't mind at all so it obviously wasn't hurting him. The acupuncturist said that he had obviously had a reaction to the vaccinations – that's where the rashes were – as well as behind his knees and elbows. Heat was being poorly transported through his body and congregating in these patches, and manifesting as rashes.

'He had two treatments. Half an hour after the first, the rashes had almost gone and after the second his skin was completely clear. Strangely, my doctor wasn't in the least bit interested about why the rashes had suddenly disappeared.'

Sandra and Joe, now 2½

RINGWORM

Ringworm is not in fact a worm at all, but a fungal infection, identified by circular scaly patches of red skin, which spread outwards and have a pronounced edge. It can appear anywhere on the body – the head, arms, nails, genital area or, as in the case of athlete's foot, on the feet. If it appears on the scalp there may be some hair loss. It is passed on from an animal or another human.

What you can do

You should seek confirmation that the condition is indeed ringworm. If on the body, let air get to the affected parts as much as possible. Discard any brushes or combs if the scalp is affected and keep the child's towels and flannels separate, to prevent spreading. Your child may be embarrassed by the bald patches and will need reassurance that the hair will soon grow back, but in the meantime they may want to wear a hat. Take any pets to the vet to see whether they are the source of the infection.

Treatment

Aromatherapy Tea-Tree oil, known for its anti-fungal properties, has been effective in treatment of ringworm. One drop applied to the area three times a day can prove beneficial. A practitioner may also recommend using Thyme which can help boost the immune system against further infection.

Herbal medicine A medical herbalist would look not only at the ringworm itself, but also at the child's general health, as, if the ringworm is widespread, it may be a sign of the immune system not being as strong as it should be. To help boost the system and treat the skin, a tea containing Echinacea, Cleavers, Wild Indigo and Yellow Dock may be suggested. Antifungal creams or lotions applied externally, such as Calendula, Marigold or Myrrh, are also helpful.

Naturopathy A naturopath would recommend keeping the skin as dry as possible. Clothes shouldn't be swopped with siblings as this can pass the infection on. Pets shouldn't be treated, too. Tea-Tree oil may be applied to the area. The immune system will need a boost to help fight off infection, so an increase in vitamins A, C, E and also zinc will be recommended. Mineral salt supplements may also be given, such as potassium sulphate and iron phosphate. To help detoxify the skin, drinking plenty of water will be advised and exercise encouraged.

Homoeopathy A homoeopath will look at the child's health and constitution and take into account how to boost the immune system to prevent further attack from infection. Sepia may also be recommended to help deal with the itchy skin.

Other therapies that may be beneficial: acupuncture.

SHINGLES

Shingles, or herpes zoster, is more likely to affect older children. If your child has a weakened immune system, for instance after illness, and they are exposed to the virus they are more likely to contract the disease. Shingles can only occur if the child has already had chickenpox (varicella-zoster). The infection attacks the nerves leading to the skin, and usually affects just one side of the body, and may cover the neck, arm and trunk. Signs of the infection include 'flu-like symptoms and extra sensitivity in the areas affected, which can become very painful. After a few days, small, red spots spreading into a rash appear which then turn into blisters. These blisters then dry out, leaving itchy scabs which eventually flake off. Some children may also suffer post-herpetic pain, or neuralgia. This sometimes intense pain is caused by damaged nerves which repeatedly send nerve impulses to the brain.

What you can do

The sooner treatment is started the better for your child, as prompt action can reduce the length of the illness and minimize the neuralgia. Try to make your child as comfortable as possible and be aware that they can be in a lot of pain. Keep them away from other children until the symptoms clear up as it is a contagious condition.

Treatment

Traditional Chinese medicine The Chinese have a pill formula called long dan xie gan wan, but this is usually kept for older children who can better stand the bitter taste. Other herbs may include Chinese Angelica and Gardenia. Externally, herbs such as Aloe Vera and Marigold may be given to soothe the skin rash and nerve pain. Acupuncture may also be given to help the skin lesions.

Reflexology A reflexologist would work not only on the area of the foot corresponding to the area where the shingles have appeared and where there may be post-herpetic pain, but would treat the whole foot to help boost the immune system.

Naturopathy The naturopath will look at the child's state of health as a whole, as conditions such as shingles tend to take hold when the immune system is already low. A diet would be tailored to help boost the immune system and may include an increase in food or supplements which contain the B vitamins which convert food into energy. Mineral salts, which help support the body's functions, such as potassium chloride, iron and sodium sulphate or magnesium phosphate, may be given. Other therapies to help relieve the pain may also be included, such as osteopathy or hydrotherapy.

Acupuncture Acupuncturists believe that we all have our weak points, and in those who suffer from shingles, it is their skin. Particular attention will be paid to the points next to the rash to help reduce the neuralgia. In Chinese medicine there are six levels of energy and shingles is seen as wind and damp heat trapped between the skin and the second level of energy. Acupuncture may help to disperse the pain and expel the virus. Daily treatment may be required early on.

Other therapies that may be beneficial: osteopathy, yoga, aromatherapy, homoeopathy, herbal medicine.

SINUSITIS (maxillary)

Sinusitis is the inflammation of the mucous membranes of the facial maxillary sinuses, the air-filled cavities around the nose, which causes pain. It usually occurs after an infection that started as a cold or sore throat spreads along the narrow passages from the nose.

Occasionally, it can also be caused by an oral infection such as an abscess, or infected water entering the nose after swimming. Mucus is unable to drain away and the tension caused by the build-up leads to pain across the face, especially when moving the head. There may also be a fever, yellow-green discharge from the nose or the nose may become blocked, leading to a loss of sense of smell. It occurs more often in older children as babies and younger children still have relatively underdeveloped sinuses.

What you can do

Monitor your child's sore throat or cold for signs of infection spreading to the sinuses. Also check that nothing has been inserted into the nose that is causing the pain. Keep the child's room moist and cool as this can help to relieve symptoms – try placing bowls of water by heated radiators, or, if your child suffers recurrent bouts of sinusitis, it may be worth investing in a humidifier. A menthol steam inhalation may also help to get the secretions moving again.

Treatment

Aromatherapy An aromatherapist may recommend a blend of oils to use during inhalation. These may include Rosemary, which has analgesic properties, Thyme, which can help fight the bacterial or viral infection, and Tea-Tree to help stimulate the immune system. Or a blend of Rosemary, Geranium and Eucalyptus may be suggested, and a drop put on a handkerchief to inhale.

Naturopathy A naturopath will ask how much dairy food is in your child's diet as an allergy may be affecting the sinuses. A diet high in citrus fruits and home-made juices may be prescribed. Epsom salts may help to detoxify and herbal medicine such as Echinacea, Golden Rod, Golden Seal and Marshmallow Leaf may be given. Supplements of mineral salts and vitamins A, B and C may be prescribed. Alternate hot and cold compresses can help to ease congestion and pressure in the sinuses.

Reflexology A reflexologist will work on the parts of the foot relating to the head as well as the adrenal gland reflex area. All of the toes will be worked on which covers the sinus cavities as well as some sensory organs, the brain, mouth and nose. Working on the areas relating to the adrenal glands will help simulate the 'fight or flight' response to help fight off infection.

Acupuncture One study found that acupuncture was successful in reducing the intensity of sinus pain in half of cases. The type of treatment will depend on whether the condition is acute or chronic. In acute cases, treatment would try to reduce the heat in the body caused by a build-up of mucus and phlegm which lead to congestion and inflammation in the sinuses. In more chronic cases, the child will be more weakened and suffer frontal headaches, exacerbated by changes in temperature and so these symptoms would be treated.

Caution

If symptoms last for more than a couple of days consult your doctor.

Other therapies that may be beneficial: homoeopathy, biochemic tissue salts, osteopathy.

'Ayleen had been suffering from headaches for about three months and was getting pain behind both her eyes. It was worse during the day, but it wasn't just concentrating on the blackboard at school, because she was bad during the holidays, too. She'd been to the doctor and had been given different things – antibiotics, anti-inflammatories and painkillers, as well as nasal sprays.

'Although the pain was better at night, she'd be coughing whenever she lay down – every thirty seconds we'd hear her. She was missing out on her sleep because of the coughing, so she'd be tired at school and quickly become exhausted after doing any sports, which she loves.

'When we went to the acupuncturist, he took her pulse and said it was very thin and rapid. He examined her tongue which I think he said was "thin and rough", and found her eyes were very red under her lower lids. I didn't know what all this had to do with her pain, but we wanted to get Ayleen better.

'I don't know what I expected, but progress was very slow. It took about fifteen treatments, but she might have got better quicker except that she caught a heavy cold halfway through which slowed her down a bit. But she's fine now – no pain and no cough, so we're all happy.'

Patrick and Ayleen, 11

SLEEPING DIFFICULTIES

Children's needs are so different when it comes to sleep, it's difficult to say what's normal and what's not. In young children, it may take a long time for them to fall into sleeping habits. And while one new baby might sleep on and off for twenty hours a day and through the night, another only naps for an hour or two at a time. Some toddlers need only one nap a day while others need two. Older children may vary their hours depending on what's happening in their life at a certain time. If your child doesn't sleep much, but is perfectly happy and coping with daily school work, then there's no need to worry. But if your child suddenly develops new night-time habits such as waking through the night, being unable or afraid to go to sleep, or starts sleepwalking, there may be an underlying problem that needs to be addressed.

What you can do

If your baby does not sleep much, get all the help you can. Take it in turns with your partner to get up during the night. Make sure there are plenty of toys or books in the cot or bed for older children to play with if they wake up. If a child has developed sleeping difficulties, try to talk to them during the day to find out if they are anxious about anything. A new sibling, troubles with a playmate, bullying at school or worries about homework may all contribute and night waking may be their way of seeking attention. Reassure your child when putting them to bed – read a cheerful story, give them a warm, milky drink and let them know you love them and are close.

Treatment

Hypnotherapy Studies have shown hypnosis to be effective in getting people to sleep more quickly. It has also been shown to have lasting effects on sleepwalkers. Hypnotherapists use the unconscious mind so the patient can learn, without being aware of learning. With sleeping difficulties this can be used to help a child go to sleep without problems and stop the need to wake during the night or to sleepwalk. A hypnotherapist is likely to try and help the child disassociate bedtime as a difficult time and instead suggest positive images of night and sleep.

Aromatherapy A warm bath, using a couple of drops of oils with relaxing and soothing qualities, such as Chamomile, Ylang-ylang or Sandalwood, just before putting your child to bed should help to calm them. A practitioner may also recommend a massage oil containing Chamomile, Mandarin or Palma Rosa, to be applied last thing at night to relax your child.

Osteopathy An osteopath may relate a baby's sleeping difficulties back to a difficult birth, when the process of labour suppressed the baby's cranial system. This can cause crying, irritability and discomfort, leading to sleeping difficulties. An osteopath may therefore work on the cranial area to relieve any pressure.

Bach Flower Remedies Children who seem quite happy during the day but become restless at night may be worried but putting a brave face on things, so a practitioner may recommend Agrimony. Open apprehension about something they can name may be helped by Mimulus, while a vague anxiety with no specific cause would need Aspen. If there is a lot of change going on in the child's life, such as a house move or a parental divorce, then Walnut may help. And Vervain would benefit those children who get so enthusiastic about things that they stay awake long after their bodies are exhausted. *Other therapies that may be beneficial: acupuncture, herbal medicine, traditional Chinese medicine.*

'I knew that hypnotherapy could work because it had helped me to give up smoking a couple of years ago. Caroline was trying to do too much at school and became very anxious about her work. She stopped seeing her friends and just wanted to keep her nose in a book every evening. She found it hard to fall asleep and then woke during the night, worrying about whatever she had to do the next day.

'But Caro was taking so long to get to sleep and then waking throughout the night, that it was beginning to affect her school-work. A couple of times she just dropped off to sleep during class. It became a vicious circle.

'She was happy to try hypnosis when I suggested it to her. The last thing we both wanted was for her to be put on sleeping pills. During the sessions, she looked back into her past and how she'd been happy at school when she had a balance between work and socializing. She responded really well and after the first session she was sleeping a lot better and had started to relax a bit about her schoolwork. She only needed three sessions in total, and now she's back to a normal outgoing schoolgirl.'

Josephine and Caroline, 11

SORE THROAT

A sore throat, where the throat feels raw and tickly and it may be uncomfortable to swallow, is usually the symptom of an infection. Coughs, colds, influenza, tonsillitis (see under relevant alphabetical sections) can all cause the throat to become sore. A sore throat is not usually a serious problem, but if it persists, consult a doctor in case of more serious infection.

What you can do

Young babies may show signs of difficulty in swallowing if their throat is sore. Babies and children may also feel generally unwell and lose their appetite. Check to see whether the glands have become swollen by running your hands down either side of your child's neck and take their temperature. Gargling with salt water may help. Give your child plenty of fluids to drink and offer easy-to-eat foods, such as soup and yoghurt.

Treatment

Herbal medicine If your child suffers from persistent sore throats and colds, the herbalist will look at ways of improving the immune system to help prevent susceptibility to further infection. They may recommend herbs that will help to boost the immune system, such as Echinacea. Herbs which work well against infection such as Indigo, Thyme and Garlic may also be given.

Homoeopathy A homoeopath will look at the child's general constitution. If they're looking flushed, have a headache and their throat is burning and it is difficult to swallow, Belladonna may be recommended. If the child's throat has been exposed to the cold, feels dry and rough and their voice is hoarse and they have a raised temperature, Aconite may also be recommended. If it hurts the child to swallow and the neck and ears are painful, leaving the child feeling weak, Gelsemium may also be prescribed.

Naturopathy A naturopath will look for the cause of the sore throat. They may feel recurrent problems could be due to a food allergy or that maybe the child's diet is too high in refined foods which are not being eliminated properly. Epsom salts to detoxify may be recommended as may a gargle, containing warm water, salt, lemon and honey or the herbal remedies Myrrh or Golden Seal. High doses of vitamin C may be advised and foods high in vitamins A, E and zinc, such as fruit and vegetables. Mineral salt supplements of magnesium and sodium phosphate may also be given.

Aromatherapy An aromatherapist may recommend using Tea-Tree and Lavender oils as both these have antiseptic properties and Tea-Tree can also help to boost the immune system. Other oils that may be used for their antiviral and antibacterial properties are Lemon, Thyme, Bergamot and Lime. The oils can be massaged in around the throat and chest area.

Other therapies that may be beneficial: osteopathy, reflexology.

SPRAINS

A sprain is the tearing or pulling of the ligaments that support the joints. It is usually caused by the sudden pulling or stretching of the joint beyond its normal limit, such as during a fall. The wrist or knee can suffer sprains, but the ankle is most commonly affected if the foot lands badly or buckles over. A sprain will cause the ligaments to bleed if torn, and swell, leaving the child bruised and in pain.

What you can do

Check to see whether the joint seems broken. If you are not sure, take your child to casualty in case an X-ray is necessary. If the knee or foot is affected, your child won't be able to put any weight on it. The affected joint should be slightly raised, so prop it up on a stool or pillows. Apply a cold compress as soon as possible to help reduce the swelling and renew every ten minutes for the first few hours and then every few hours.

Cover the area with thick wads of cotton wool and bandage up the sprain, by binding carefully, but not too tightly, in figures of eight.

Treatment

Aromatherapy An aromatherapist may recommend a foot-soak, for instance using Sweet Marjoram, known for its anti-inflammatory and analgesic properties, and Rosemary, which works well for conditions such as sprains that suffer spasmodic pain. Add a couple of drops of these to a bowl of cold water and soak the affected joint for fifteen minutes. A cold compress may also be made up using the same solution and be held in place with clingfilm.

Homoeopathy Arnica may be recommended by a homoeopath to help halt the swelling and reduce the pain as well as the feeling of shock. This may be followed by Rhus tox., if the pain is due to a fall and the joint feels stiff and painful. Bellis perennis also works well on swollen and painful ligaments, particularly if they occur on the left side of the body.

Reflexology If a foot was sprained, a reflexologist would not try to work on it, but would use pressure on the hand instead, relating to the injured area. Treatment would include helping the child deal with the shock and anxiety they may be feeling after a bad fall. Work would be gentle so that the area does not become overstimulated.

Chiropractic A chiropractor would recommend that if a fracture or dislocation has been ruled out, then rehabilitation of the sprained joint should begin as soon as possible. They may recommend passive mobilization for the first few days to prevent the joint from stiffening. They may use mobilizing and manipulative techniques according to the joint affected and supervise the introduction of rehabilitative exercises to restore the function of the injured joint. The child should only put pressure on the joint and soft tissue work should only be started once there is no risk of disrupting any inter-muscular bleeding or injured ligaments.

Other therapies that may be beneficial: osteopathy, acu-puncture, acupressure, biochemic tissue salts, Bach Flower Remedies.

'We went to a chiropractor because Michel had fallen and sprained his knee, which didn't seem to be getting better as quickly as it should. But he'd been having problems with his knees for about nine months, particularly the right one. Both of them would ache and had given way on a couple of occasions in the previous two weeks. He said his left ankle also hurt and that he had had cramp in both calves in the last couple of months.

'I was worried that there may be some underlying problem and, as I'd read a bit about chiropractic, decided to try it. Even so, I was really surprised by what the chiropractor said. It seems his pelvis was misaligned which was the root of all his problems and meant he was not getting the support in the right place.

'He had three treatments to realign the pelvis and after that both knees were fine, although his ankles still ached sometimes when he got up in the morning.'

Jean-Paul and Michel, now 15

STRESS

We tend to think of only adults as suffering from stress, but children are just as susceptible to physical and emotional stress factors. The arrival of a new sibling, starting primary school, end-of-term exams, parental divorce, boyfriend troubles can all lead to stress and worry for a child. Stress can manifest itself in a number of ways, such as bad behaviour, lack of concentration at school, bullying. Or it may be the trigger of a physical illness, such as asthma, eczema or diarrhoea. The child may also become depressed and withdrawn.

What you can do
If you know a certain event, such as a new baby or starting a new school, is going to prove traumatic, take early steps to reassure your child. Don't give your child too long to think about a distant event, but near the time, start positively preparing them for the changes that are to come. For any problem that may be causing your child stress, try to talk it out with them and work out ways to minimize the cause of the stress, or how it may be better handled.

Treatment
Hypnotherapy Hypnotherapy uses methods which will help the child to unconsciously learn, without being aware that they are learning. The unconscious mind can cope with a lot more than the conscious mind and so can help your child to learn to deal with stress. This may be done by recalling when stress was dealt with in the past and had a positive outcome and learning how to use that knowledge in the future.

Bach Flower Remedies Depending on the cause of the stress, the child may be given any number of remedies. If the child is feeling rejected in any way, Larch will help with the feelings of lack of confidence and low self-esteem. Cerato may work well if they are feeling vulnerable and need reassurance. If there is jealousy over a new sibling, Holly will help to relieve those feelings, and Chicory will help the selfishness and the feeling of being left out.

Reflexology A reflexologist will use different techniques depending on why the child is stressed, for instance, as a result of an injury, how they are handling the stress, how long they have been suffering and so on. The big toes which relate to the head will be particularly worked on, but the whole foot may be covered, according to the child. Apart from this, the one-to-one attention they will be receiving and a listening ear will also be a great help.

Aromatherapy There are many oils that can have a calming, soothing effect on children. An aromatherapist may recommend a blend of oils, added to their bath or used in massage, depending on the cause of the stress. Chamomile Roman can help soothe the nerves and relieve insomnia, if the child is lying awake, worrying. Geranium can help depression and nervous tension and if stress results in a physical ailment, such as eczema. Used in small amounts (otherwise it acts as a stimulant), Lavender can relax and bring the emotions back into balance.

Other therapies that may be beneficial: Alexander Technique, herbal medicine, homoeopathy, osteopathy.

SUNBURN

A child's skin is a lot thinner and more sensitive than an adult's, allowing higher levels of UV (ultraviolet) rays to penetrate, leading to burning. Studies have shown that even one incidence of burning when young can increase the risk of skin cancer when older. There are two types of harmful UV rays.

UVB rays are the strong summer rays which penetrate the skin's outer layer, the epidermis, and stimulate the production of melanin, the brown pigment that gives us a tan. This pigment protects our body against harm, but when overworked, the skin burns. This can lead to skin cancer as well as attacking the skin's suppleness.

UVA rays are present throughout the year. They are

more powerful than UVB rays as they penetrate deeper into the skin's layers, down to the dermis, causing longer-term damage. These rays attack the skin's fibres, causing dryness and possibly skin cancer.

What you can do

The best remedy for sunburn is to prevent it. No child should be in the sun long enough to allow them to burn and children under a year old should not be exposed to the summer sun at all. If your children are going out in the sun, especially if abroad, always apply a sunscreen that gives both UVA and UVB protection and avoid the hottest part of the day. Look for products that contain high sun protection factors (SPF), such as SPF15, and also look out for products that carry the star system, which gives the UVA protection factor. Four stars (★★★★) give the highest protection.

Liberally apply any creams, oils or lotions before letting your child go into the sun, reapply hourly, always reapply after swimming and even when the sun's heat lessens in late afternoon. Don't forget sensitive areas such as the eyelids, ears, lips and nose. Make sure your child wears a wide brimmed hat and t-shirt when they have had enough sun, and use a buggy parasol.

Treatment

Herbal medicine Aloe is used extensively in over-the-counter remedies for soothing the skin after sun exposure. But a herbalist would recommend the real thing – the leaves with their medicinal gel – applied directly to the burn, as this will be a lot more beneficial. Marigold may also be recommended as a useful anti-inflammatory, as can Myrrh. Fresh cucumber juice and dock leaves placed on the burn may also bring relief.

Homoeopathy Belladonna may be recommended by a homoeopath as it works well for the pain and burning on the skin associated with sunburn. Apis may also be used if the burning is accompanied by fever.

Bach Flower Remedies If the child is feeling sore and obviously in distress, Rescue Remedy cream should help with minor sunburn.

Caution

Look out for signs of heatstroke (caused by the body's normal heat-regulating system malfunctioning) if your child has been exposed to a lot of sun, as it can be fatal. Symptoms of over-heating include a raised temperature (up to 104°F or 40°C), hot, dry skin, lethargy and drowsiness, fast pulse, confusion. The child may also lose consciousness. Lie the child down in a cool place, check their pulse and temperature and cool the body down with tepid (not cold) water and fan them. Give plenty of fluids. Consult a doctor or take your child to casualty immediately if their temperature reaches 104°F, 40°C.

TEETHING

Teething can be a difficult time for both parent and child, as the first, or primary, teeth move through the jaw and start to come through the gums. This begins at around six months, with usually the front top or bottom teeth coming through, followed by the others. Most teeth will have come through by the time the child is about three years old. Although teething won't cause a problem during all of this time, there will be periods when your baby produces more saliva and dribble, will constantly push their fingers or other objects into their mouths or chew them. Your child will probably become more fretful and irritable, will wake more often during the night and the cheeks may look flushed and swollen.

Other ailments such as diarrhoea, vomiting, nappy rash,

raised temperature, loss of appetite, ear ache or coughing are often attributed to teething but if your child is suffering from any of these always check with your doctor or practitioner.

Secondary, or permanent teeth come through at about six years of age. The permanent back molars grow in addition to the primary ones, while at the front of the mouth, the teeth loosen and drop out and new ones then gradually emerge.

What you can do
Teething is not a serious problem, although it can make everyone more irritable if you've had a few sleepless nights in a row. But the reason your child is being grizzly is probably because they're in discomfort or pain. Keep patient and give them lots of attention. There are plenty of products available, such as teething rings, which can also be put in the fridge to bring cool relief to gums. Or you can give your child raw apple or carrot to chew on. If your child has lost their appetite, give cool, easy-to-eat foods such as ice-cream or jelly.

Treatment
Homoeopathy A homoeopath may give a variety of remedies, depending on the child and their symptoms. If the child is restless and nervous, Actaea may be given, or Chamomilla if they are irritable, clingy and want to be held all the time. If the child seems to be in a lot of pain and have a raised temperature, Aconite may be recommended. If the child is very fretful, Colocynth. Biochemic tissue salts such as Calc. phos. may be given as it is said to help strengthen teeth and bones and is particularly good if the teeth are late in coming through. Or Combination R, which uses more than one of the tissue salts, may be recommended by the homoeopath.
Herbal medicine There are some gentle herbs that may be given by a herbalist to help relieve the pain of teething. Peppermint has cooling properties to help soothe the

inflamed gums, while the mildly sedative effects of Chamomile can help to calm the child down and act as an anti-inflammatory.

Bach Flower Remedies Depending on how your baby is reacting to teething, a number of remedies may be recommended by a practitioner. Impatiens may be given for a child who has short-tempered irritability and Cherry Plum for the screaming tantrums. Children who are clingy and don't want to be put down may be helped with Chicory. Walnut is also helpful at times of change, including those that happen to the body, such as teething.

Naturopathy A naturopath may give the homoeopathic remedies of Chamomilla and Aconite or the herbal remedies of Meadowsweet tincture or Marshmallow Root. Mineral salt supplements, which can help to support the body's functions, such as calcium, magnesium and iron phosphates, may be recommended. The naturopath may try to soothe your child by massaging Lavender and Chamomile oils into the abdominal area or gently smoothing them on to the cheek.

Other therapies that may be beneficial: aromatherapy, reflexology.

'Sammy was a very quiet, placid baby until he started teething at about six months old. He'd been healthy, happy and had no problems at all, but the teething really seemed to affect him. His mouth was obviously really sore and he'd dribble all day, which made his chin sore, too. His urine became very acidic which made his nappy rash worse and made that area very uncomfortable for him. Not surprisingly, I suppose, he became very fractious and irritable.

'I'd been going to a medical herbalist myself, so when he got bad, I took him along, too. I didn't like the thought that he probably still had months of this before all his teeth came through. I was given a chamomile infusion for him to drink to help calm him. Then an infusion of chamomile and peppermint which I had to rub on his gums. Peppermint has wonderful cooling effects and he always calmed down and seemed happier once I'd given it to him. I wouldn't say it worked every time he got really grouchy, but it did help.'

Gaynor and Sammy, 11 months

THRUSH

Thrush or *candida albicans*, is a fungal infection which can occur in babies' mouths or in the nappy area, particularly the anus. It's caused when the fungus which normally lives in natural balance in the intestines with other bacteria, proliferates, causing infection in the gastro-intestinal tract. This tends to occur when the natural balance is upset by the use of antibiotics, or if your child's immune system is low after illness. If the mouth is affected, you will see small white patches covering the inner cheeks, the top of the mouth and tongue. Unlike similar looking milk patches, it is difficult to rub off these patches or they may leave raw, bleeding areas underneath. Thrush in the genital area may look like nappy rash, but will not respond to the usual treatment.

What you can do

Giving live yoghurt will help to bring the body's natural bacterium back into balance. Change the nappies regularly and immediately after passing stools to minimize the spread of infection. Keep the nappy off and leave the area exposed for as long as possible. Stick to mild foods that are easy to swallow until the infection has cleared up and avoid all sugary and yeasty products.

Treatment

Naturopathy If thrush has developed after taking antibiotics, a naturopath may recommend supplements such as acidophilus and bifidus to help replace the useful bacteria in the body. Other causes may be food sensitivities or excess fruit juice. Stress can also play a part as this depletes the body of vitamin C and the B vitamins, leaving an environment where the fungus can thrive. So a diet high in vitamins A, B, C and E may be prescribed and supplements such as mineral salts.

Homoeopathy A homoeopath may recommend Borax for oral thrush. For genital thrush, Mercurius or Rhus tox. may be given if the skin is very itchy and blisters have formed.

Herbal medicine For oral thrush, a herbalist may recommend a Calendula tincture, which has antiseptic and antifungal qualities, and can help to stimulate the immune system to fight off infection. For the nappy area, Calendula or Marigold cream may prove effective if gently rubbed on the area. A herbalist may also recommend mixing a little Myrrh tincture into the Marigold cream to help recovery and advise Echinacea to help boost the immune system.

Aromatherapy If your child suffers from oral thrush and is old enough to rinse with a mouthwash without swallowing, an aromatherapist may recommend swilling a combination of well-mixed Tea-Tree and Myrrh oils in a glass of water. Tea-Tree has great antifungal and antiseptic qualities and will also stimulate the immune system to combat infection, while Myrrh can work particularly well against oral infections. Massaging oils such as Tea-Tree, Chamomile, Lemon and Thyme into the nappy area will also help to relieve the discomfort and soothe.

TONSILLITIS

Tonsillitis is the inflammation of the tonsils which are at the back of the mouth. The tonsils are there to help protect the upper respiratory tract from becoming infected, but can be susceptible themselves to bacterial or viral infection. Symptoms include a sore throat, enlarged and red tonsils which may be covered in little yellow spots, difficulty in swallowing, a raised temperature and sometimes bad breath. The adenoids may also become enlarged. The child may also get ear ache and suffer temporary deafness.

Tonsillitis is common in children over a year old and can be a recurrent problem, although most grow out of it by the age of nine or ten.

What you can do

If your child complains of a sore throat, feeling unwell and has difficulty in swallowing, check for tonsillitis by tilting their head back, pressing down the tongue with the handle of a clean spoon and asking them to say 'ah'. This will open up the throat to enable you to see any signs of enlargement or infection. Make sure they get plenty of rest, drink lots of fluids and give them food that is easy to eat, such as soup or yoghurt and drinks containing lemon and honey to help cleanse and soothe the throat.

Treatment

Aromatherapy Oils can be massaged around the neck, throat and chest area, or applied in a compress. Tea-Tree oil is known for its antiviral and bacterial qualities as well as being a useful antiseptic. Lemon is also a good antiseptic and can help to fight off infection. Ginger can be used for many ailments and can help combat catarrh, which can develop as a result of infection. Lavender, Chamomile, Sandalwood and Thyme all also have healing properties which can help against the infection. A therapist may recommend four drops of any of the oils mixed thoroughly in a bowl of warm water and applied as a compress, or five drops of oil to 2fl. oz (56ml) of carrier oil, such as Sweet Almond, massaged in, which should help to bring relief.

Homoeopathy A homoeopath will ask which side of the throat is most affected before deciding on treatment. If the right side seems worse, and if the child has fever, the tonsils are very swollen and red, and the neck stiff, Belladonna may be prescribed. If the left side is affected and swollen and it hurts for the child to swallow, Lachesis may be prescribed. If the child suffers recurrent bouts, and the glands are enlarged and tender, Baryta Carb. may help reduce the symptoms.

Naturopathy A naturopath will look for possible causes, such as what they see as excess mucus linked to a diet high in mucus-forming foods such as dairy products and low in vegetables. A fruit diet might be recommended for up to three days and Epsom salts given to help detoxify. High doses of vitamin C may be advised and vitamin A as beta carotene can help to clear mucus. A gargle of warm water, salt, lemon and the herbal remedies Myrrh or Golden Seal may be beneficial and a throat compress of Mullein given. Also, a throat wrap using tepid water on a cotton cloth wrap for an hour at a time can help to stimulate healing by increasing circulation and lymph flow in the area.

Herbal medicine A herbalist will work on boosting the immune system as a whole, as it is when it is weak that infection such as tonsillitis sets in. Gargling with a mouthwash of Sage, Wild Indigo, Thyme or Myrrh, which all have antiseptic and stimulating qualities, may be recommended.

Other therapies that may be beneficial: osteopathy, traditional Chinese medicine, acupuncture.

'David had a mild case of tonsillitis. It wasn't too bad, but it still made him grumpy and uncomfortable. I know there's not too much you can do with the illness, except plenty of bedrest and drinks to sip, but I felt I wanted to relieve it a bit if I could.

'I went to my aromatherapist and explained his symptoms to her. She made up a blend of Eucalyptus, Lavender and Chamomile mixed in a white lotion to smoothe on around his throat. She said the Eucalyptus can help relieve infection, while the Lavender can help to dull the pain and acts as an antiseptic and Chamomile is a natural anti-inflammatory.

'I applied it regularly to David's throat and within a couple of days he was feeling a lot better and ready to eat more solid food.'

Noa and David, 7

TOOTHACHE

Toothache is usually caused by a tooth decaying or as a result of a tooth fracturing. The ache can be caused by one or more of the teeth and sometimes the gums. Tooth decay is caused by plaque, which contains saliva, food and bacteria which all make up an acid that erodes away the surface of the tooth, until the nerve is exposed. Eating hot, cold or sweet food can all affect the sensitive nerve, triggering pain. Other dental problems may also develop, such as abscesses (see *Abscesses*), bad breath or peritonitis, when the tissues surrounding the root of the tooth become inflamed.

What you can do
Toothache is often a sign that a tooth is already in an advanced stage of decay. The best way to prevent both toothache and decay is by making sure your children brush

their teeth properly. One of the main culprits in the decay is sugar and the longer it sits in the mouth, the more harm it does. Try to restrict sweet food to mealtimes. Make sure children brush their teeth twice a day and rinse well to make sure all the toothpaste is removed. Dental floss should also be used regularly to clean in between the teeth.

Babies should not be left with bottles of milk or juice to fall asleep with, as this can stay in the mouth when the child drops off, leading to early decay. Try to encourage young children to brush their teeth from the earliest possible age. Children should be taken to the dentist for check-ups every six months from when they have their first full set of teeth.

Treatment

Naturopathy A naturopath will look for the cause of the toothache. It may be due to the child grinding their teeth, in which case stress factors will be looked at and supplements given, such as mineral salts, calcium and magnesium phosphate and vitamin B5. If decay is causing pain, your child's diet will be looked at – too many refined foods and commercial juices high in sugar can lead to decay. A diet high in fresh organic foods with plenty of fresh fruit and vegetables would be recommended, with water or home-made fruit juices to drink.

Bach Flower Remedies Children who seek constant attention would need Chicory, while those who feel sorry for themselves would take Willow. Tiredness might be a problem if the toothache stops the child from sleeping properly and for this Olive may be indicated.

Homoeopathy If the pain is on one side, and is aggravated by cold wind, a homoeopath may recommend Aconite. If the child is very irritable with the pain, which becomes worse at night, Chamomilla may help, or Silicea if the pain is also aggravated by hot or cold food. If the child has had a filling, Arnica may bring relief.

Traditional Chinese medicine Apart from decay, TCM sees toothache as either heat in the stomach and large intestine's channels or as an attack of wind cold in the stomach and spleen. A mouthwash containing Ginger, Cloves and Cinnamon with Sweet Flag may be given. For acute toothache, a paste of crushed garlic may be placed on the acupuncture point relating to the tooth, which is left on for two hours, although it is warned this can blister the skin.

Biochemic tissue salts A homoeopath or other practitioner may also recommend the use of these salts. Calc. phos. may be advised for decaying teeth and also teething problems.

Other therapies that may be beneficial: aromatherapy, reflexology.

TRAVEL SICKNESS

Travel or motion sickness is quite common in children and those aged between three and twelve are thought to be particularly susceptible. It can happen if the child is travelling by any means of transport – car, plane or boat, or even a rollercoaster. It is caused when the minute balance mechanism in the inner ear is upset by repetitive movement. The eyes become accustomed to motion, but the ears do not and it is the resulting confusion of messages to the brain that can trigger symptoms.

Symptoms may be mild, such as a feeling of queasiness and discomfort to severe distress, vomiting, feeling faint and sweating.

What you can do

The best way to help your child is to try and prevent the sickness, rather than treating it. Try the following tips.

- Avoid giving them a full meal before travelling.
- Keep the car windows slightly open so the air doesn't become stuffy.
- Keep any food out of sight, as this may trigger queasiness.
- A child who has been sick once is more likely to be sick again, so keep reassuring an anxious child before a journey. Let them know it's all right to be sick and they should try and give warning so you can stop the car.
- Don't give them books or comics to read while travelling, so they aren't continually looking down and then up, as this can also be a trigger. Play games where they have to focus on something on the horizon.
- Wrist bands which work on the Chinese principle of acupressure by pressing on the point of the wrist which controls nausea are available from chemists and are drug-free. There are also brands that contain drugs which may cause drowsiness.
- Give the child a ginger biscuit or a piece of root ginger to nibble on as this reduces nausea.

Treatment

Acupressure Press three fingers' width in from the inside wrist crease, massaging in a circular motion for a few minutes, putting the pressure towards the centre of the wrist. Studies have shown the effectiveness of acupressure in reducing symptoms.

Homoeopathy If the practitioner knows your child suffers from motion sickness, they can prescribe remedies for you to take on any trips. If your child feels worse when they smell food, begin to salivate and wants to lie down, Cocculus may be recommended. If they feel nauseous, dizzy and want to eat a little something, Petroleum may be better. If air travel is a particular problem, especially on landing, Borax may work well.

Aromatherapy A couple of drops of oil on a tissue which can be inhaled during a journey can be helpful. Ginger is well known for helping quell nauseous symptoms. Other oils which may help are Bergamot, which can aid the digestive system, and Orange, known for its calming properties.
Other therapies that may be beneficial: reflexology, naturopathy, Bach Flower Remedies.

ULCERS (mouth)

Children often suffer from ulcers, although girls tend to be more susceptible than boys. They're also more likely to occur if other members of the family have them. The most common type are *aphthous* ulcers, which occur singly or in clusters on the tongue, gums, inner lips or cheek and can be caused by stress, allergies, or sensitivities. They are small, roundish and look grey, yellow or white with an inflamed edge. Other types of ulcers occur as a result of an injury, such as biting the soft mucous membrane of the tongue or inside of the cheek, or when a toothbrush fibre has pierced the gum. Some blisters that look like ulcers may be cold sores or thrush (see under relevant alphabetical section). Ulcers will heal on their own, but this can take up to a couple of weeks and can be very uncomfortable for the child.
What you can do
If your child seems to have difficulty in eating or has lost their appetite due to discomfort or complains of a sore mouth, check for ulcers. If your child suffers from recurrent ulcers, check with your doctor for any underlying cause. Give your child easy-to-eat foods, such as yoghurt, and steer clear of salty or spicy foods as these can aggravate the condition.

Treatment

Naturopathy Stress factors can cause an imbalance in the metabolism, according to naturopaths, and so increase acidity, leading to mouth ulcers. To combat this a low fruit, high vegetable diet should be recommended, as fruit is high in acidity. To help boost the immune system, supplements such as zinc, vitamin A as beta carotene, vitamins C in an alkaline form and E may be given. Plenty of rest is advised, water to help detoxify and the child should avoid sharp foods such as crisps.

Herbal medicine Hops have long been used for ulcers for their antiseptic qualities. A herbalist may also recommend using parts of the Ginkgo Biloba tree, which works as an astringent and stimulant. Giving a liquorice stick to chew may also be a pleasant way to help speed up the healing process. However, too much can have a laxative effect. A mouthwash using an infusion of Sage or Thyme may also be given, but only if the child is old enough not to swallow it.

Aromatherapy If your child is old enough to use a mouthwash without swallowing, a therapist may recommend rinsing with water containing an essential oil such as Tea-Tree to help speed up the healing of the ulcers. Tea-Tree oil has known antiseptic qualities and can also help to stimulate the immune system, as ulcers often set in when this is low. A couple of drops well mixed in a cup of cooled boiled water should help. Other oils that may aid healing are Lemon, Geranium and Thyme.

Kinesiology A practitioner will look at the possible causes of the immune system becoming weak and at ways of supporting it. They may also advise a diet that is high in the vitamin B complex and vitamin E, and that salty and sweet foods are avoided while the ulcers remain.

'A friend of mind is a kinesiologist and she suggested I take my daughter to see her, who's always suffered from mouth ulcers, to see if she could find out the reason why.

'Fran is very confident and outgoing, but she puts herself under pressure about being good enough and worries about things underneath, without letting on. Claire, the kinesiologist, said that because she was feeling tense and stressed she might not be creating or absorbing enough of the B vitamins from the small intestines, so that the mouth ulcers kept recurring, especially when she felt low.

'Claire worked on balancing her endocrine system and supporting the immune system and recommended taking B-complex and vitamin E every few days. Soon after the mouth ulcers went completely and Fran hasn't had any since.'

Helen and Fran, 7

URTICARIA (hives/nettle rash)

Urticaria is an allergic reaction when the skin erupts into itchy raised white wheals, surrounded by red inflammation. The wheals are caused by the body releasing histamine. These may appear in small patches, or cover large areas of the skin, anywhere on the body. The condition is not usually serious and the wheals tend to disappear within seventy-two hours. Other symptoms may include fever, fatigue and nausea.

Certain types of food are known to cause an allergic reaction in susceptible children which can trigger urticaria. Common allergens are milk, strawberries, shellfish, onions, beans, nuts, potatoes, spices, and food additives, particularly tartrazine (E102). Other known triggers are insect stings or bites, some plants, penicillin, mould, animal dander, aspirin and even bacterial or viral infections.

Susceptibility to urticaria can disappear in due course, but for some, repeated exposure to the allergen can make the condition chronic.

What you can do

Try to be aware of any foods or other triggers that cause your child to break out in hives. Avoid any known allergens as much as possible and alert your child's school, if you feel it is necessary. Keep the area cool and apply Calamine lotion to relieve the itching. Adding three tablespoons (45ml) of sodium bicarbonate to relieve the itching, or a cupful of vinegar, to the bath may help calm the skin down.

Treatment

Naturopathy If your child is allergic to aspirin, they may also be allergic to foods that contain salicylates, a natural compound used in aspirin. So a naturopath may suggest trying to cut down on foods high in salicylates, such as most fruit, particularly dried fruit and berries, a variety of herbs and spices, liquorice and peppermint. In lower levels, salicylates can also be found in nuts, seeds, fish, pulses, grains, dairy products, meat and vegetables. No elimination diet should be followed without careful supervision and, unless the urticaria is a repeated problem, it is probably not necessary.

Homoeopathy A homoeopath may recommend Urtica Urens or Apis which will help to relieve the itching, particularly if the wheals are sensitive to touch. If your child suffers a particularly acute reaction, Aconite may be advised.

Herbal medicine To treat the actual itching, a herbalist may recommend an infusion of Chamomile, to help relax the child and soothe the inflammation, or Chickweed which can help to relieve irritation and can also be applied as an ointment or poultice. An Aloe Vera gel will also soothe the area, particularly if mixed with a Chamomile cream.

Osteopathy An osteopath will work to try and boost the immune system by decreasing the mechanical strains in the body. This may be done through cranial work to enable the release of more energy to fight off disease and to improve the interchange of fluid between tissues, for instance blood and lymph fluids.

Caution

If urticaria develops in or around the mouth, seek immediate medical attention as it may cause swelling of the tongue or throat and lead to breathing difficulties.

VACCINATION

For some parents, the question of whether or not to give their child the government-recommended vaccinations is a sensitive one. Most children suffer no side-effects after their vaccinations. But there are a small number that do. Vaccinations are given from the age of about two months onwards:

2 months:	1st Diphtheria, Tetanus, Whooping Cough, Polio, Haemophilus Influenzae b (Hib)
3 months:	2nd Diphtheria, Tetanus, Whooping Cough, Polio, Haemophilus Influenzae b (Hib)
4 months:	3rd Diphtheria, Tetanus, Whooping Cough, Polio, Haemophilus Influenzae b (Hib)
12–18 months:	Measles, Mumps, Rubella (MMR)
4–5 years:	Diphtheria, Tetanus, Polio
15–18 years:	Diphtheria, Tetanus, Polio

Other immunizations such as BCG will also be given at around twelve or thirteen years old.

Parents should be warned by GPs and health visitors

about the small number of children who will react badly to the vaccines, suffering convulsions, paralysis or brain damage. But there are lesser side-effects from allergic reactions to personality changes (happy, placid child to irritable, uncontrollable child) that have affected some children, and in the case of the MMR (measles/mumps/rubella) vaccine, some parents have reported language difficulties and sensory distortions.

What you can do

Get as much information as you can on the vaccinations your child is to receive. Talk to your doctor or health visitor about any concerns you may have. Your child should not be immunized if they are suffering from an acute illness until they are better, if they have had a severe reaction to a previous vaccination, or are taking any medication that might affect their ability to fight off infection. They do not have to have the vaccinations at the recommended times, nor do they have to have the combined jabs.

Treatment

Homoeopathy Homoeopathic treatment can be effective to counteract vaccination side-effects and can be given before and/or afterwards. Treatment will depend on the vaccination given and the type of side-effects.

Osteopathy An osteopath would work to help increase the child's own immune system to deal with the vaccine entering the body. This may be done by mainly working on the lymphatic system and to rebalance any effects of the vaccine.

Traditional Chinese medicine A TCM practitioner may recommend leaving vaccination until as late as possible to allow the child's own defensive energy to develop. TCM sees a *mild* reaction to a vaccination, such as mild fever, restlessness and difficulty in sleeping, as a good sign as it shows that the vaccine 'has taken' and that the body's Qi or vital energy is strong. Tonic herbs such as Ginseng and Chinese Angelica, or acupuncture, may be given before a vaccination to help the child's constitution. Herbs may also be given as part of aftercare to help clear the phlegm that often tends to build up after vaccination.

VERRUCA

(See *Warts*)

VOMITING

There can be many reasons for your baby or child to be sick, or vomit, when the contents of the stomach are forcibly brought up through the mouth. It is very common for young babies to projectile vomit occasionally, and in such cases no treatment is necessary. In some cases, it may just be over-excitement or over-indulging on too many sweets that turns their stomachs and is nothing to worry about. But there can be other causes that need closer attention, particularly if the vomiting is accompanied by other symptoms. If your child vomits for more than six hours, consult your doctor immediately. Common causes of vomiting include:

- regurgitation: this occurs when a baby regurgitates or possets some milk after feeding, usually when burping. This is quite normal.
- pyloric stenosis: projectile vomiting (sometimes shooting out by a few feet) in babies around eight to twelve weeks old. This is caused by the thickening of the pyloric muscle which controls the movement of food out of the stomach. Treatment is usually necessary with drugs or surgery.

- food intolerance: your child may be intolerant or allergic to milk products (see *Allergies*).
- coughs and colds: the force of coughing can make a child vomit and if the child is swallowing a lot of mucus this can sometimes also cause vomiting (see *Coughs* and *Colds*).
- food poisoning/gastroenteritis: other symptoms include diarrhoea, raised temperature and loss of appetite. Call for medical assistance if symptoms last more than six hours, because of the risk of dehydration (see *Food Poisoning*)
- infection: other symptoms may include fever, headaches, loss of appetite and possibly spots or rash (see *Fever, Measles*).
- meningitis: other symptoms may include severe headache, dislike of bright light, lethargy, drowsiness, stiff neck and sometimes a rash (see *Meningitis*).
- travel sickness: any motion such as air, car or boat travel can set off nausea and vomiting (see *Travel sickness*)
- migraine: other symptoms include flashing lights, abdominal pain and numbness in the affected part of the head (see *Migraine*).

What you can do

Always monitor your child if they are vomiting, even if it is only due to too many sweets, as it can lead to dehydration. Make them comfortable and have a towel in front of them and a bucket nearby to be sick into. Give frequent, small sips of liquid. To help prevent dehydration, give frequent cups of water with a pinch of salt and a teaspoon of sugar added. Give only bland foods and avoid milk until the stomach settles.

Look out for any other symptoms and signs of dehydration, which include a dry mouth, depressed fontanelle in babies, sunken eyes, listlessness, and call for medical assistance if you are in the least bit worried.

Medical attention should be sought if the vomiting lasts longer than six hours, but the following complementary therapies may also be beneficial:

Treatment

Naturopathy Vomiting is a sign that the body is ridding itself of unwanted matter or toxins and a naturopath will look at possible causes for this before treatment. Warm abdominal compresses may be given and ginger tea and white toast recommended once the symptoms have eased. Simple foods such as brown rice and vegetables should be given slowly. Probiotics, such as acidophilus and bifidus or live yoghurt will help to replace healthy flora in the bowel. Mineral salt supplements such as potassium chloride, iron, sodium, calcium, potassium or magnesium phosphates may also be given.

Herbal medicine Ginger is a well-known remedy for vomiting. A herbalist may recommend giving your child some root ginger to chew or recommend an infusion of a teaspoon of grated ginger root in a cup of boiling water which should be strained and cooled before drinking. Chamomile and Peppermint tea will help, as Chamomile is calming and relaxing to the digestive system and helps to stimulate digestive function while Peppermint has the effect of soothing the bowel and helps prevent wind forming. Meadowsweet may also be recommended for its abilities to soothe the lining of the digestive tract. It can help reduce acidity and calm feelings of nausea. Other herbs that may be recommended include Catmint, Fennel, Lavender, Dill and Cinnamon.

Bach Flower Remedies A practitioner may recommend remedies that can help treat the emotions that can accompany vomiting. Guilt would be eased with Pine, while any feelings of distaste, shame of uncleanliness would be removed with Crab Apple. Crab Apple is also useful to help the body cleanse itself. If stress or anxiety is a contributory factor, a number of remedies may help, depending on the child's nature. Vervain would help the over-active enthusiast, while Mimulus is for the shy, timid child and Rock Water for the perfectionist whom demands too much of her/himself.

Traditional Chinese medicine Chinese medicine sees vomiting as a food blockage, especially in children under three, cold in the stomach and spleen or heat in the stomach. Signs for heat in the stomach will include a red face, sweating, constipation, loud cries and smelly vomit. Cold signs will include a pale face, diarrhoea, cold sweats, pale vomit containing undigested food. Generally, Ginger will be given to help calm the stomach, but other herbs will be given, depending on diagnosis. A practitioner will always advise seeing a doctor if the symptoms don't improve quickly with TCM.

Caution

Seek medical attention if your child vomits for more than six hours because of the risk of dehydration. To help prevent dehydration, regularly give your child a cup of water containing a pinch of salt and one teaspoon (5ml) of sugar to sip.

Other therapies that may be beneficial: naturopathy, acupuncture, osteopathy.

'Frank had been vomiting from birth, but I actually took him to see a TCM practitioner because his breathing was very gurgly and I was worried as asthma runs in our family.

'He was always sick about an hour or two after a feed, when his milk would come up again, watery and curdled. I mentioned that his forehead seemed sweaty after feeding and his tummy was distended. He suffered terribly from constipation – only going every three or four days and becoming more irritable the longer it went on – and then he was obviously in pain when he did move his bowels.

'She diagnosed a food block which was making his stomach's "energy force" rebel, which she said was also creating phlegm in his lungs and causing his gurgling noises. She said she had to treat the bowel problem first and gave him herbs and acupuncture to clear the food blockage and stagnation. Then he had herbs to strengthen the stomach and lungs.

'Now he has daily bowel movements and has stopped vomiting, even when he moved on to solids. And as yet, there are no signs of asthma.'

Sue and Frank, now 18 months

WARTS

There are many different types of warts, which are caused by a contagious virus, but are usually pretty harmless. They are small lumps with a rough surface of dead cells that can appear anywhere on the body, such as the face, hands, legs or on the soles of the feet, when they are known as verrucae. They sometimes have black dots, which are clotted blood capillaries. As they are contagious, they are easily passed on by children, who may get one or more on different parts of the body.

What you can do

Warts may disappear many months after their arrival without any treatment. But you may want to remove them if they are in a place where contact means they can be passed on to others. The verruca virus, for instance, is easily picked up in places where it thrives such as the warm, moist conditions in showers and swimming pools.

Treatment

Hypnotherapy The power of the unconscious mind over matter seems to work in the case of warts. One study has shown that warts on the hands or feet were significantly reduced on those who were treated with hypnotic suggestion compared to those who weren't.

Homoeopathy There are many different remedies that may be able to help, depending on the type of wart, although Thuja is often used. But the homoeopath will treat the child constitutionally so that the immune system is strengthened and can fight off infection rather than treating the wart itself.

Herbal medicine Rubbing garlic on to the wart is an old remedy that many have found useful, but you should protect the surrounding skin with Vaseline. A tincture containing Thuja will help the warts, particularly if used in conjunction with the homoeopathic Thuja tablets. Vitamin C may also be recommended to help boost the immune system.

Other therapies that may be beneficial: aromatherapy, traditional Chinese medicine.

WHOOPING COUGH

Whooping cough, or pertussis, mainly affects children and is particularly serious in babies under a year old. Symptoms include long bouts of coughing, when the child expels air from the lungs, followed by a 'whoop', the sound made as breath is rapidly drawn again. Whooping cough is a contagious disease, spread by airborne droplets which lead to inflammation of the upper respiratory tract. Newborn babies are particularly vulnerable as they have not sufficiently developed the technique of drawing in breath. The bouts of harsh coughing can lead to vomiting in some children.

There is an incubation period of one to three weeks and

the whooping cough itself can last for ten weeks or even longer. It begins with 'flu-like symptoms of sneezing, mild coughing, runny nose, fever and aching limbs. The coughing which in most, but not all, cases ends with the 'whoop' then becomes worse, particularly at night. Complications such as pneumonia can arise and the vomiting should be monitored in case of dehydration.

The number of cases of whooping cough have dropped in recent years. But in the 1970s, fears of side-effects such as seizures or permanent brain damage led many parents to stop vaccinating their children. But it is again on the increase (see *Vaccination*). If a child has any history of seizure, a progressive neurological disorder, has had a previous reaction to vaccination or is ill at the time, vaccination should not be given.

What you can do

If your child has whooping cough, keep them warm and well rested. Give plenty of fluids. If they are vomiting a lot, keep a bucket and towel nearby and give frequent cups of water with a pinch of salt and a teaspoon of sugar added to help prevent dehydration. Give small snacks to eat after vomiting as they are more likely to keep food down then. During a coughing attack put a bowel under their chin to spit phlegm into. Don't give cough suppressants.

A baby may need to be kept in hospital under observation to prevent dehydration and to monitor for any signs of other infection.

Treatment

Osteopathy To help deal with the effects of whooping cough, treatment may include working on a number of areas, such as the spine, ribs and diaphragm to help improve the mechanics of the chest, lung function and lymphatic drainage and combat scar tissue in the lungs. Exercises may also be recommended to help improve breathing and advice given on posture.

Traditional Chinese medicine This illness is seen to come in three stages. The first twenty days is a normal cough, the next forty to sixty days the child will have the characteristic whoop and will cough until they vomit. At this stage other problems can set in such as asthma and a weakened stomach. The third stage lasts one to six months when the entire system is weak, known as Qi Xu. The Chinese believe that whooping cough in younger children is a sign of underlying food blockage and if this is treated quickly, recovery can be fast, although there may be set-backs. A mixture of herbs will be recommended for the phlegmy cough. Patients may also be given Fritillaria and loquat syrup which is said to be helpful.

Homoeopathy A homoeopath may recommend Drosera if your child's throat is dry and tickly, they fight for breath between coughs and vomit after coughing hard. If the coughing is worse at night, the child vomits up stringy mucus and is helped by sipping water, Coccus may help to bring relief. If the coughing is worse in the early hours of the morning and the cough is a dry, hacking one, Kali carb. may be recommended. If the mucus coughed up is yellow and stringy, Kali bichrom. may help.

Caution

Seek medical help immediately if you think your child may have whooping cough.

WORMS

There are many different types of worm, but the most common in the UK is the threadworm. These are usually ingested in unwashed fresh fruit and vegetables contaminated with the worm eggs. These then hatch in the intestine, growing into adults after about twenty-eight days. The female worms then lay eggs around the anus, usually at night, causing itching. If your child then scratches around the anus area and his or her hand later goes into the mouth and the eggs are swallowed, the cycle begins again. Eggs can live for up to three weeks in bedding. Symptoms include itching around the anus, white thread-like worms in the stools or around the anus.

There is also the toxocara worm which lives in the intestines of cats and dogs and can be passed on to children if they happen to touch the egg-infested animal's faeces and then their mouth, leading to the toxocariasis infection. The eggs hatch and the worms then tunnel through the intestinal wall and into the bloodstream. The cycle begins again if they are coughed up from the lungs and then swallowed. Symptoms include fever, loss of appetite, bouts of abdominal pain and, in rare cases, sight can be affected.

What you can do

In the case of threadworms, if your child seems to be scratching, inspect the area, particularly at night, or check your child's stools for signs of the thread-like worms wriggling about. The whole family may need to be treated as the worms or their eggs can easily be passed on. Always make sure food is thoroughly washed before serving.

In the case of the toxocara worm, try to ensure that any pets defecate well away from where your children play. If going to parks, try to prevent children eating grass if dogs are not controlled. Encourage your child to always wash their hands after touching animals or playing in the garden. Regularly worm your pets.

Over-the-counter anti-worm medication can seriously upset digestive balance, leading to abdominal pain and digestive weakness. So, if possible, alternative remedies such as homoeopathy should be tried first.

Treatment

Homoeopathy A homoeopath will look at the child's general health and hygiene and may recommend, in the case of threadworms, Cina for the intense itchiness at night. If the itchiness is causing lack of sleep at night and the child has become irritable, Teucrium may be recommended.

Naturopathy A naturopath would encourage a balanced diet, as a diet high in sugar, dairy and meat will have a lowered resistance to worm infestation. A weak digestive system is also less resistant to infection, so problems such as constipation will also need to be looked at. A diet high in fruit and vegetables and low in meat and sugar will be recommended, as well as drinking plenty of water. Mineral salt supplements may be given and eating garlic and cayenne pepper will help stop reoccurrence as worms don't like these. Herbal remedies such as Wormwood, Senna, Capsicum and Quassia may also be recommended.

Traditional Chinese medicine A Chinese practitioner may recommend you give your child onion and garlic as worms hate these. Pumpkin and melon seeds may also be advised as well as plenty of fresh fruit and vegetables and less sugar and refined foods. A variety of herbs may be given, but as these can taste very bitter (to the worms, too) they may be ground up and made into a capsule rather than given as a drink.

Other therapies that may be beneficial: aromatherapy, herbal medicine.

Section II

The Therapies

ACUPRESSURE

Anyone who has ever suffered a headache or sinus trouble and has found some relief by putting gentle pressure on the area that is causing pain has tried acupressure in its simplest form. But the actual training of acupressure is a lot more complex.

Acupressure has been in use for thousands of years, and was a feature of all the great Oriental medical traditions. Pressure and massage are used with usually the fingertips on various points along the body's meridians – invisible or electrical – channels. It is believed that these meridians carry the energy or life force, known as Qi (pronounced chee) through the body. Mental, physical, emotional and spiritual health is balanced by the opposing but complementary forces of *yin* and *yang*. When these forces become imbalanced, then illness or dis-ease follows. Pressure on points along these meridians help to restore the life force and so health. Traditional Chinese practitioners believe there are 365 points along the 14 meridians, but more modern practitioners have found up to 2000 points to help treat every ailment. See drawing opposite for some of the principal points used.

How the therapy works

As with acupuncture, once diagnosis has been made, pressure is put on certain points along the body. This can vary in combination and from light touch, such as in Shen Tao, to firm pressure, such as in Shiatsu, depending on your child's problem. Your child may be asked to lie on a mattress or padded table and pressure will be exerted, with the fingers and thumbs, or sometimes hands, elbows, knees or feet. It may be slightly uncomfortable, but shouldn't be painful.

Light acupressure can easily be used at home. If you are

EXAMPLES OF ACUPRESSURE POINTS

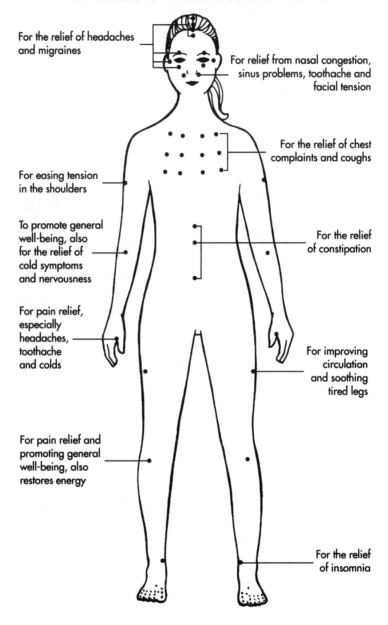

For the relief of headaches and migraines

For relief from nasal congestion, sinus problems, toothache and facial tension

For the relief of chest complaints and coughs

For easing tension in the shoulders

To promote general well-being, also for the relief of cold symptoms and nervousness

For the relief of constipation

For pain relief, especially headaches, toothache and colds

For improving circulation and soothing tired legs

For pain relief and promoting general well-being, also restores energy

For the relief of insomnia

EXAMPLES OF ACUPRESSURE POINTS

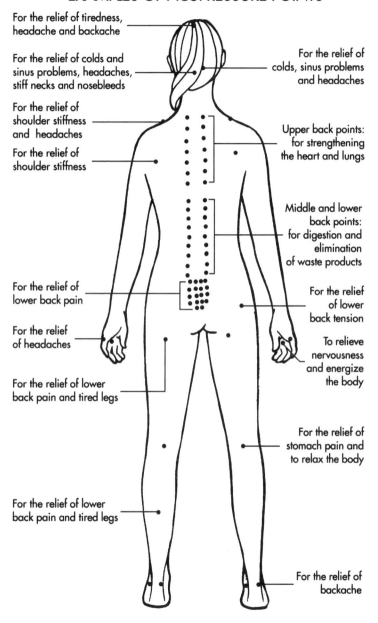

For the relief of tiredness, headache and backache

For the relief of colds and sinus problems, headaches, stiff necks and nosebleeds

For the relief of shoulder stiffness and headaches

For the relief of shoulder stiffness

For the relief of colds, sinus problems and headaches

Upper back points: for strengthening the heart and lungs

Middle and lower back points: for digestion and elimination of waste products

For the relief of lower back pain

For the relief of lower back tension

For the relief of headaches

To relieve nervousness and energize the body

For the relief of lower back pain and tired legs

For the relief of stomach pain and to relax the body

For the relief of lower back pain and tired legs

For the relief of backache

treating your child at home, make sure they are warm and relaxed before you start. If you are not sure of their ailment, always consult a doctor or practitioner before applying any pressure.

What to expect from a first visit

A practitioner will first discuss your child's condition and why you have come. Detailed notes will be taken, including general health, family medical history, personality traits, diet, bowel movements and so on, to build up an overall picture. They will then look at your child's tongue, seen as a strong indicator of overall health, checking its colour, texture and coating. The Chinese believe there are twelve pulses, six on each wrist, which relate to the energy of the body's organs and functions and these will also be checked. Pressure will then be applied to the appropriate points. This may take around forty-five minutes.

Finding a therapist

The practitioner should be trained to the same high standard as an acupuncturist (see below) and training should include anatomy, physiology, pathology and diagnosis. Always ask the practitioner what experience they have of treating children as this is a specialist field and experience is advisable. Personal recommendation is also one of the best methods of finding a therapist. For a list of practitioners, contact:
Shiatsu Society, 31 Pullman Lane, Godalming, Surrey GU7 1XY. Tel: 01483 860771
Shen Tao Foundation, Middle Piccadilly Natural Healing Centre, Holwell, Sherborne, Dorset DT9 5LW.
Tel: 01963 23468.

Qualifications

Many practitioners – those trained in acupuncture, Shiatsu, Shen Tao and so on – practise acupressure, so the qualifications will vary (see also under Acupuncture).

Use with other therapies

Other therapies, such as the Alexander Technique, osteopathy, chiropractic and Chinese herbal medicine may all work well with acupressure, depending on the ailment.

Any dangers

Acupressure can be safely used at home for problems such as headaches and stress. However, overstimulation can temporarily make the symptoms worse. Rather than just trying pressure on sore points, it is better to gain guidance from a qualified practitioner or use a good book. If you are in any doubt about your child's symptoms, always consult your GP. Certain points are contraindicated during pregnancy.

How much will it cost

A first consultation may be around £25, depending on which area of the country you live in.

Availability on the NHS

Not specifically available, but may be used in conjunction with acupuncture.

Helpful reading

Acupressure Techniques Dr Julian Kenyon, Thorsons
Acupressure for Common Ailments Chris Jarmey and John Tindall, Gaia

ACUPUNCTURE

Acupuncture has been in use by the Chinese for around 3500 years and has also been extensively developed in Japan and Korea for many centuries. Its exact origins are not known, but some believe that its power was first noticed when soldiers who had been shot by arrows, not only survived, but were also cured of other long-standing ailments. Others feel the system was developed gradually by Taoists with deep awareness and sensitivity to subtle energy. It was an oral tradition, passed on from family to family and was first put in written form around 3000 BC. With each passing Chinese dynasty, techniques in its use have been developed, leading to a complex system of medicine. It lost some popularity during the Ch'ing dynasty (1644–1912) when Western medicine became more widespread. Acupuncture is now widely used again in China and the rest of the world, including the UK. The first edition of the medical journal *The Lancet*, in 1823, reported its use in treating rheumatism.

The basis of Chinese philosophy is that health depends on the flow of Qi (pronounced chee) or vital energy. This is not just your child's physical health, but mental, spiritual and emotional. This constantly moving flow travels around the body via invisible channels, or meridians. The flow depends on the perfect balance of the opposing yet complementary forces of *yin* and *yang*. They are always changing, as day turns into night, spring into summer, but Yin is perceived as the

ACUPUNCTURE MERIDIAN CHANNELS

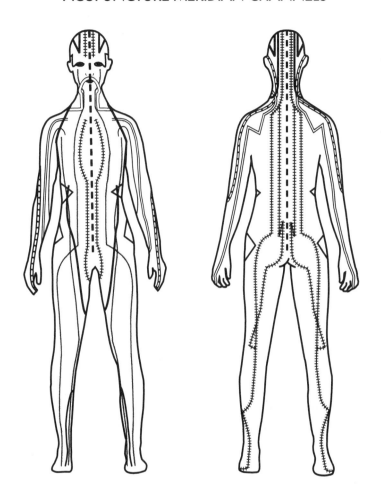

KEY TO THE MERIDIANS

—————— lung and large intestine	▬▬▬▬ heart governor and triple heater
┷┷┷┷┷ stomach and spleen	╌╌╌╌╌ gall bladder and liver
—————— heart and small intestine	┅ ┅ ┅ governing vessel and
══════ bladder and kidney	conception vessel

female force and represents dark, cold, passive and negative, while Yang is the male force, light, warm, aggressive and dry. They also correspond to different parts of the body. Yin organs are dense and blood-filled such as the liver and heart. Yang organs deal with absorption or discharge in the body, such as the stomach and gall bladder. If there is an imbalance between yin and yang, when one becomes deficient (or excessive), the energy flow becomes stagnant or blocked and the Chinese believe this leads to illness and disease (or dis-ease). This imbalance can be caused by stress, unhealthy diet, anger, drugs or the environment.

How the therapy works

It is the role of the acupuncturist to identify the imbalance and redress it by inserting needles at appropriate points on the body. There are 14 meridians or channels that run through the body, seven each of yin and yang. Along these there are traditionally 365 pressure points, although modern acupuncturists believe there are up to 2000. By inserting the needles in the right points after diagnosis, the Qi should be released to flow freely again, restoring good health. This can also be done with acupressure or shiatsu massage, which uses pressure rather than needles. See accompanying drawing outlining the meridians for reference.

Moxibustion may also be used when it is felt the patient needs more energy and heat. The same acupuncture points are used, but the herb moxa is burnt (on a stick, cone or needle) and applied to the point. It heats the skin but doesn't burn.

Acupuncture is also commonly used with Chinese herbs as part of traditional Chinese medicine (see below). A combination of herbs may be prescribed, which usually have to be boiled and then drunk.

What to expect from a first visit

Expect a long first consultation of about an hour, although subsequent visits will be a lot shorter. The acupuncturist will need to build up a detailed picture of your child before diagnosis. This will involve questions about why you have come, your child's general health, family medical history, their personality, likes and dislikes, what they like to eat, their bowel movements, how they form part of the family and so on. They will then examine the child's tongue. The Chinese see the tongue as a great indicator of health. Its colour, texture and shape can reveal much about deficiencies. Your child's pulses will be taken on both wrists – there are twelve in Chinese medicine – to gauge the energy of particular organs. Only then will diagnosis be made.

Fine sterile needles will then be inserted into the appropriate points. The needles should be sterilized according to procedures set out by the Department of Health.

In adults, the needles are usually left in for a few minutes. But with children this is obviously more difficult if they won't keep still, and as they also generally respond more quickly to treatment the needles are inserted, gently manipulated for a few seconds and then withdrawn. The child may feel a slight sensation, but it should not hurt, although the surprise may make them cry. Young children tend to have four to six points used at each session, while older children may have more. Most children don't seem to mind the fine needles and it is the parents who may be more anxious, but acupressure or a stimulator pen can be used if it is a problem.

The total number of treatments will depend on your child's illness and how they respond, but may be anything from one or two to about eight. If there is no change after at least five sessions, you should maybe think again about treatment.

Finding a therapist

Most acupuncturists who have undergone comprehensive training in this country are now members of the new umbrella body, the British Acupuncture Council. The Council sets guidelines for codes of practice, ethics, discipline, training and education.

The acupuncture profession is also moving rapidly towards statutory recognition following in the footsteps of chiropractors and osteopaths. This will mean that, in the near future, only those with the appropriate qualification will be able to practise. Always ask the practitioner what experience they have of treating children, as this is a specialist field and experience is advisable. If you can, reinforce your choice of practitioner with personal recommendation. To get a list of acupuncturists who are BAC members, contact:

British Acupuncture Council Park House, 206–208 Latimer Road, London W10 6RE. Tel: 0181 964 0222

Some doctors have also trained in acupuncture, but it is worth finding out how long that training actually lasted for. For a list of acupuncture-trained doctors, contact:

British Medical Acupuncture Society Newton House, Newton Lane, Lower Whitely, Warrington WA4 4JA. Tel: 01925 730727

What qualifications to look for

As a member of one of the above organizations, the acupuncturist should have had a training of two to four years and have medical insurance. Being a member of the

British Acupuncture Council means they must abide by their standards. Training includes qualifications in anatomy, pathology, physiology and diagnosis. There is also specialist graduate training available in paediatric acupuncture. Look for letters following their name, such as DipAc (Diploma of Acupuncture), LicAc (Licentiate in Acupuncture) or BAc (Bachelor of Acupuncture). Also look for the letters M or F, denoting them as a member or fellow of one of the former organizations which is now the BAC, eg FBAAR. All members of the newly formed British Acupuncture Council should now use the new designation MBAcC in place of the old initials. Check if your practitioner has this qualification.

Use with other therapies

Acupuncture can be used with many other therapies, although it is always advisable to consult your practitioner. It is often worked in conjunction with traditional Chinese herbalism and also works well with chiropractic, osteopathy and the Alexander Technique.

Any dangers

Although the head, neck and chest are potentially danger-ous areas, acupuncture with a trained practitioner should pose no danger at all, as the fine, sterilized needles need not penetrate deeply. In the event of teenage pregnancy, advise the therapist, as certain points can induce labour. If you are in any doubt about your child's symptoms, always consult your GP.

How much will it cost?

Many therapists will charge lower rates for children, but it is up to the individual practitioner. Expect to pay around £25–£35 for the first visit and less for subsequent ones. Acupuncture is now covered under many private health insurance schemes.

Availability on the NHS

Acupuncture is now more widely available on the NHS, with some doctors happy to refer on, while others practise it themselves. It is also becoming more popular as a method to treat pain in hospitals, particularly since it was discovered that acupuncture can stimulate the release of endorphins and enkaphalins, the body's natural painkillers.

Helpful reading

Introductory Guide to Acupuncture Dr Paul Marcus, Thorsons
Principles of Chinese Medicine Angela Hicks, Thorsons

AROMATHERAPY

The use of essential oils derived from plants to help heal the mind and body is many centuries old. The Egyptians pressed flowers to make medicine around 600 BC. The ancient Persians used water from distilled roses to help treat illness. And in the eleventh century, the Arab philosopher and physician Avicenna developed the method of distillation to produce a more pure form of essential oils, and the Crusaders brought the idea back to Europe.

Since then aromatic oils have been popularly used down the centuries for their healing properties, for cosmetics and for perfumes. The oils are found in the tiny glands of petals, leaves, stems, wood, berries and bark and give plants and trees their powerful aromas, particularly if crushed. But in the nineteenth century, the pure oils were copied with cheaper, chemical versions, which led to a decline in their popularity. But now the pure essential oils have made a comeback in an age when the benefits of nature are being sought once again.

The resurgence started at the beginning of the twentieth century when French chemist René Gattefosse accidentally burned his hand at the family's perfume house and soothed it by covering it with Lavender oil. He noticed how quickly the burn healed without blistering or scarring. Gattefosse went on to document his findings and the therapeutic use of other oils. His work was followed up by other French nationals, Dr Jean Valent who treated war wounds and other conditions such as TB, cancer and emotional problems; and the bio-chemist and beautician Marguerite Maury, who developed the use of oils for massage and beauty treatments.

Today, the use of essential oils is well known and well documented. Aromatherapy provides a holistic, non-invasive method for improving emotional and physical health by preventing, as well as treating, illness. There have been numerous world-wide studies into the efficacy of oils to treat a wide range of illnesses, physical, mental, emotional and spiritual. Aromatherapy is used widely in the UK in hospitals and establishments such as hospices by midwives, nurses and practitioners for many conditions. Many patients attest to the benefits in reducing stress and anxiety which accompany many serious problems.

Many oils have particularly beneficial therapeutic qualities. For instance, Tea-Tree oil, which comes from the Australian marshlands, is stronger than many artificial antiseptics, yet is totally harmless. It has antibacterial, antiviral and antifungal properties and can also help to boost the immune system, making it an invaluable natural remedy. Lavender is also well known for its medicinal qualities. A shrub that grows in many countries, it is also a natural antiseptic as well as a mood balancer, analgesic, antibiotic, and sedative and helps the cells to regenerate more quickly, making it particularly useful for skin problems.

How the remedies work

Many people still view aromatherapy as a nice smelly massage. But science has shown that essential oils do have a proven positive effect on us. For instance, it is believed that Lavender increases the alpha rhythms in our brains which induces calmness.

Aromatherapy is not just used in massage, although this is the most common form of use. Massaging means the oils penetrate the skin and are absorbed into the bloodstream, dispersing their effects through the body. But their scent can also be inhaled in a bath or a bowl of hot water, which is said to have an immediate effect on the brain. They can also be used in vaporizers, compresses and mouthwashes (if the child is old enough not to swallow).

Therapists say there are no side-effects (except, if relevant to a teenage girl, during pregnancy) and that even young babies can benefit from aromatherapy.

What to expect form a first visit

An aromatherapist should take a detailed account of your child's general health, medical history (including any medication taken), family background, lifestyle, likes and dislikes. This may take about an hour. The information will enable them to choose the right oils to suit your child and be aware of any contraindications to certain oils. The aromatherapist will then blend the appropriate oils which may be used in massage or be given for inhalation, a compress, or vaporizer. They may also give you a blend to take for home use (see p.217).

Depending on the ailment, only one session may be needed, but for more chronic problems, a course of treatment may be necessary. If a course is needed, the blend of oils will change according to the child's physical and emotional progress.

Finding a therapist

Always ask the practitioner what experience they have of treating children as this is a specialist field and experience is advisable. Personal recommendation is also one of the best methods of finding a therapist. There are many different organizations in the UK which train aromatherapists. In 1991 the Aromatherapy Organization Council was formed as a governing body to unify the profession and set up common standards of training. Member organizations of the AOC must provide training which includes 180 hours in class involving 80 hours of aromatherapy, 60 hours of massage and 40 hours of anatomy and physiology. For a list of member organizations contact:

Aromatherapy Organizations Council (AOC) 3 Latymer Close, Braybrooke, Market Harborough, Leicester LE16 8LN. Tel: 01858 434242

What qualifications to look for

There are over ninety training establishments recognized by the AOC. If you contact an aromatherapist who has trained at one of these establishments they should be of a standard acceptable to the AOC and abide by their Code of Conduct and Ethics.

Use with other therapies

Aromatherapy works very well on its own, but can be used successfully with other therapies. Therapies that work on the body, such as reflexology, osteopathy, chiropractic and applied kinesiology can all gain from the added benefits of aromatherapy. Avoid use with homoeopathy as the strong scents can disturb the homoeopathic remedies.

Any dangers

Used properly, essential oils are very safe. If your therapist gives you oils to take for home use, they should warn that the oils are not to be taken internally, as they are potent. Unless otherwise stated, they should always be diluted with a carrier oil. If you are in any doubt about your child's symptoms, always consult your GP. Some oils are contraindicated for babies and young children and during pregnancy.

How much will it cost

Sessions cost from about £20.

Availability on the NHS

Aromatherapy is widely used within the NHS. Midwives may use it on newborn babies with colic, nurses practise it on children staying in hospital for chronic conditions and to relieve the stress of an enforced stay. However, it does depend on the particular hospital, as each will have its own policy and some are more open to complementary therapies than others. However, it is unlikely that your GP will refer you directly for treatment on the NHS.

Helpful reading

Aromatherapy for Babies and Children Shirley Price and Penny Price Parr, Thorsons
Aromatherapy for Mother and Baby Allison England, Vermilion

BACH FLOWER REMEDIES

Bach Flower Remedies may not be as well known as some of the other complementary therapies or remedies, but its advocates are numerous and worldwide.

The power of the Bach Flower Remedies is in their essence. Flowers have a wonderful effect on people in their colour, scent and touch. They can influence the emotions and the mind, as anyone who has walked through a heady rose garden can tell you. It is these qualities that the Englishman Dr Edward Bach developed into a system of healing that is now used throughout the world.

Born in 1886, Dr Bach qualified as a physician in 1912 and went on to become a bacteriologist, immunologist and homoeopath. But he gradually found himself becoming more interested in the patients themselves rather than their illness. He realized that the basis of many physical ailments lay in emotional imbalances, and that every person's emotional outlook affected their physical health. He believed that to bring back a natural equilibrium, the person as a whole should be treated, not just the ailment. And the key to equilibrium was in nature.

So in 1930 he gave up a very successful Harley Street practice and moved to Wales to concentrate on developing a natural method of healing that would treat the person rather than the disease, would be easy to use and caused no side-effects.

Over the next six years he explored the English and Welsh countryside for the right plants. He would concentrate on a particular emotion, often going through it himself, such as lack of confidence, jealousy, hopelessness or apprehension and search for a plant that would help that emotion.

Eventually he found all the flowers that were needed. He believed that dew on the flowers contained their energizing properties and it was this he collected. However, he soon found he could not collect enough dew for the demands of his patients and found that floating the flowers on spring water in sunlight achieved the same results.

He developed thirty-eight remedies, for every mood, emotion and personality. He put these under seven headings: disinterest in present circumstances, apprehension, uncertainty and indecision, loneliness, over-sensitivity to influence and ideas, despondency and despair, and over-concern for others. Taken on their own or in combination they cover every state of mind and so can help everyone, whatever their ailment.

Dr Bach claimed his set of remedies were complete, and the Bach Centre maintains this stance. But there are also now many other types of flower remedies being made around the world, such as the Australian Bush Remedies and Pacific and Hawaiian remedies.

How the Remedies work

Because the Remedies treat the cause rather than the effect, every child, whatever their ailment, can be treated. Although they can't cure an illness such as mumps directly, they can help the child on the road to recovery and can be used alongside conventional treatments. Each remedy is given depending on the characteristics of your child. You'll need to think about personality and emotional states rather than the illness itself.

So for a child who is often travel sick, rather than treating the sickness itself, you will treat the anxiety, worry or mental tension that might be causing the sickness. Or to help a child recover from measles, you will have to look at how they've dealt with the illness. For example, are they impatient to get better, or have they lost interest in the outside world. Scientific studies of the Remedies show that they contain nothing but water and alcohol, although it has been said that tests so far are just not sophisticated enough to detect the energy of the Remedies. And there are many ready to claim their benefits.

What to expect from a first visit

The therapist will need to learn as much about your child's character as possible. They will need to know their likes and dislikes, how they react to certain situations, whether they are outgoing or shy, contented or anxious, have a happy or sad disposition and so on. Don't be surprised if some odd questions are asked, even those seeming totally irrelevant will have a purpose in building up a picture of your child's character.

These sort of questions are asked by most complementary therapists, such as homoeopaths, acupuncturists and so on as part of their general consultation and may take up to an hour.

Finding a therapist

Practitioners who use the Bach Flower Remedies may also specialize in other fields and use the Remedies in conjunction with their own therapies. But they will always give Bach Flower Remedies alone if that is what you ask them for. Always ask the practitioner what experience they have of treating children as this is a specialist field and experience is advisable. Personal recommendation is also one of the best methods of finding a therapist.

To find a practitioner in your area, contact the Bach Flower Centre. The Remedies can also be used successfully at home with no side-effects (see p.220). There are many books available that can help a parent to choose the right Remedies. *The Dr Edward Bach Centre* Mount Vernon, Sotwell, Wallingford, Oxford OX10 0PZ. Tel: 01491 834678

Remedies can be obtained from most health food shops or by mail order from:
c/o Nelsons Pharmacy 73 Duke Street, London W1M 6BY. Tel: 0171 495 2404

What qualifications to look for

All the practitioners listed by the Bach Centre have been trained at the Centre itself and have signed a Code of Practice and Ethics. Look for the phrase 'Registered with the Dr Edward Bach Foundation'.

Use with other therapies

Bach Flower Remedies are successfully used with other therapies, such as reflexology, acupuncture, homoeopathy and herbal medicine. They do not interfere with these therapies.

Any dangers

The remedies are perfectly safe to use. If you are in any doubt about your child's symptoms, always consult your GP.

How much will it cost

Buying the Remedies yourself will cost £2.75 per stock remedy. They are available from most health food stores and larger chemists. A therapist will incorporate the cost into their general consultation.

Availability on the NHS

Not specifically, but may be used as part of other therapies. GPs may also write a prescription for them.

Useful reading

Growing up with Bach Flower Remedies Judy Howard, C W Daniel
The Twelve Healers and Other Remedies Edward Bach, C W Daniel
The Bach Flower Remedies Step by Step Judy Howard, C W Daniel
The Encyclopaedia of Flower Remedies Clare Harvey and Amanda Cochrane, Thorsons

BIOCHEMIC TISSUE SALTS

Only in natural balance can we attain perfect health, believe complementary practitioners. And one of these practitioners, a German homoeopathic physician, Dr Wilhelm Schuessler, believed that ill-health could be caused by an imbalance of natural minerals that the body needs.

In the 1870s he developed what he termed the biochemic tissue salts. He produced twelve tissue salts, which could be taken easily in a tablet that melts in the mouth, would be quickly absorbed and would restore a healthy balance.

Although scientific research has shown that our bodies do contain at least twelve tissue salts, doctors would not necessarily argue that a deficiency of these is the cause of some illnesses.

How the remedy works

Each tissue salt has properties which can help ailments such as coughs, colds, sore throats, hayfever and headaches.

The tissue salts are prepared in the same way as homoeopathic remedies and are highly diluted. The usual potency is 6x, which is one part of the salt mixed with nine parts lactose (milk sugar) and then the process is repeated six times. However, unlike the homoeopathic treatment which works on the basis of like treating like, the salts work by restoring the mineral deficiency which is believed to be causing the illness.

What to expect from a first visit

Your child may be prescribed biochemic tissue salts as part of their treatment by a naturopath, homoeopath or herbalist (see under relevant therapy).

Finding a therapist

You won't find a therapist whose work solely involves the tissue salts. You are more likely to be seeing a homoeopath, naturopath or herbalist who will use the remedies as part of their treatment. Always ask the practitioner what experience they have of treating children as this is a specialist field and experience is advisable.

Biochemic tissue salts are very useful for home treatment under the guidance of your therapist.

What qualifications to look for

As you will be seeing a naturopath, homoeopath or herbalist, you should check the relevant qualifications needed for practising these therapies (see under relevant therapy).

Use with other therapies

Biochemic tissue salts can be used with most other therapies, without interfering with their treatment. Homoeopaths, naturopaths and herbalists regularly use the tissue salts as part of their treatment.

Any dangers

The salts are non-toxic and not addictive. Children with lactose (milk sugar) intolerance may be allergic to the tablets. The tissue salts should not be used instead of seeking professional medical advice or that of a practitioner. If you are in any doubt about your child's symptoms, always consult your GP.

How much will it cost

The price of the tissue salts may be included in the price of the consultation of the naturopath, homoeopath or herbalist. (See under relevant therapy for cost guide.)

Availability on the NHS

None, unless used by a practitioner such as a homoeopath.

CHIROPRACTIC

From its development around one hundred years ago, chiropractic has grown into a modern-day treatment that is now only third to conventional medicine and dentistry. Chiropractic uses hand manipulation to work on the body's muscles, joints and particularly the spine. The term comes from the Greek, 'cheiro' meaning hand, and 'praktikos' meaning practical action. Although the art of manipulating the muscles and joints has been around for many centuries, it was Dr David Palmer who, in 1895, established chiropractic as we know it today. He believed that if vertebrae of the spine were not moving correctly then this could not only affect the immediate muscles and nerves causing local pain but also cause nerve interference creating pain in other parts of the body, such as the arm and leg, for example, sciatica. Also less obviously related problems, such as bedwetting, sore throats, colic and constipation could be caused in this way.

Dr Palmer's first patient was the office janitor who had gone deaf after he had bent down and heard a click in his back, many years before. He allowed Dr Palmer to examine him, who found a stiff bone in his neck and manipulated it. The janitor's hearing was restored. Although a rather extreme example of how chiropractic can work, it is now a popular form of treatment for musculo-skeletal problems. There have been many studies into its efficacy and many doctors are happy to refer patients on if they feel chiropractic may be able to help the patient.

Chiropractic works very successfully on children – their

spines are more flexible, so they tend to respond to treatment far quicker than adults. A difficult birth, breech baby, long and arduous labour or use of forceps can all affect the delicate spine in a newborn, leading to colic, crying and sleeplessness. And although these may disappear, problems may develop later in life. As children learn to walk, tumbles and falls may all cause the spine damage and as they grow older, badly designed chairs and desks at school can aggravate any problems. The problems may not be obvious, but there may be signs such as persistent ear ache, interrupted sleep or stiffness in the neck, indicating that vertebrae in the spine are not functioning well.

How the therapy works

Many people confuse chiropractic with osteopathy. Although they both manipulate joints, chiropractors tend to use X-rays more in diagnosis and may also arrange for blood and urine tests. Once diagnosis has been made, varying techniques will be used to try to treat the problem and correct any stiff joints. For babies and young children, only light fingertip adjustments need be made. For older children, the chiropractor may use a combination of heavy or light thrusts in quick and shallow movements, depending on your child's condition. The joints and muscles may also be massaged to relax the child.

What to expect from a first visit

To help make his or her diagnosis, the chiropractor will need to build up a detailed history of your child. Questions about your child's birth, medical history, previous complaints, general lifestyle, how they play and sit will be asked. Their

posture and way of walking will be analysed and a full examination of the spine performed, looking out for stiff and
painful joints and muscle spasm, and checking for any nerve
impairment. Rarely, an X-ray may also be taken and blood
and urine samples may be needed to back up their diagnosis.

Actual treatment might not begin until the second visit.
This will involve your child stripping down to their underwear and standing, sitting or lying. Then, depending on the
condition, the chiropractor will mobilize or rotate the spinal
joint within its normal range of movement. They will then
make a rapid thrust to the vertebra, pushing it just beyond its
normal range and a 'click' may be heard. This helps to relax
the muscles that control the joint which have been in spasm.
Normal mobility should then be returned. Although the
quick movements may come as a surprise to the child, they
shouldn't hurt. But the area may feel a little sore for a while.
Some exercises may be given to do at home.

Finding a therapist

Up until now there has been no Government regulation for
chiropractic in the UK and standards have been set by reputable, but voluntary, organizations (see below). But now a
General Chiropractic Council is being set up which will gov-
ern standards in education, practice and code of conduct for
all chiropractors. The GCC will open a register on which
only fully qualified chiropractors can enter. Always ask the
practitioner what experience they have of treating children as
this is a specialist field and experience is advisable. Personal
recommendation is also one of the best methods of finding a
therapist.

British Chiropractic Association Equity House, 29 Whitely
Street, Reading RG2 0EG. Tel: 01734 757557

The British Association of Applied Chiropractic (BAAC) The Old Post Office, Cherry Street, Stratton Audley, Nr Bicester OX6 9BA. Tel: 01869 277111
McTimoney Chiropractic Association (MCA) 21 High Street, Eynsham OX8 1HE. Tel: 01865 880974

What qualifications to look for

Members of the BCA must have a BSc degree, gained after a full-time five-year course at a recognized training college and have a postgraduate diploma after working for one year at a clinic. This means they should have BSc DC after their name.

Members of the BAAC should have DC (WSC) or (OCC) after their name and members of the MCA should have MCMMCA or MCAMCA, depending on whether they are full or associate members. (The MCA qualifications are currently under review, so for future reference, check with the association.) They will have to have completed an intensive four-year part-time course and spent a year working in a clinic. These members do not use X-rays in their diagnosis, but will refer you to your GP or local hospital.

Use with other therapies

Although it is probably unnecessary to combine chiropractic with other manipulative treatments such as osteopathy, many therapies such as aromatherapy, herbalism and homoeopathy can complement its treatment.

Any dangers

A fully qualified practitioner should know exactly what they are doing and which techniques can be used on a child, and when it is appropriate to do so. Babies will be handled, of course, with particular care. If you are in any doubt about your child's symptoms, always consult your GP.

How much will it cost

First sessions may cost around £30–£40, but may be up to 50 per cent cheaper for children, depending on the chiropractor. An additional charge may be made for an X-ray (around £10–£25). Subsequent sessions will be much less. Chiropractic treatment is also now available under many private health insurance schemes.

Availability on the NHS

Numerous studies have proved the effectiveness of chiropractic on a number of complaints and it is now widely accepted as a bona fide form of treatment by those in the medical profession. Many GPs are happy to refer their patients on to chiropractors and some fundholding GP practices may pay for certain treatment.

Helpful reading

Introductory Guide to Chiropractic Michael B. Howitt Wilson, Thorsons

HERBAL MEDICINE

Herbs are the forerunner of modern medicine and indeed many drugs given today are derived from them. They have been used since primitive man first foraged for plants to survive and for many centuries food and medicine were one and the same thing.

There are many ancient documents purporting to the use of herbs. There survives a papyrus dating from 1500 BC in Thebes which details many herbs, such as cinnamon, still used today. The Greek physician Hippocrates, who is known as the father of medicine and was born around 460 BC, wrote a list of over four hundred herbs. And the Greek philosopher Aristotle, born in 384 BC, put together one of the first records on the use of herbs on the body.

The Roman invasion of Britain brought many herbs to this country and centuries later, as explorers set out to discover the rest of the world, more were brought back.

The popularity of herbs grew and herbalists began to set up their own shops or apothecaries. One of the most famous of these was Nicholas Culpeper (1616–54) who, in 1649, wrote *The English Physician Enlarged*, which is still in print. And one of the first established herbal firms, founded by Henry Potter in 1812, still exists today. Herbs became available from Europe, the Americas, the Middle East, Asia, and India as well as China. But with the growth of modern medicine came the decline in popularity of herbal medicine. It became thought of as a 'quack' treatment, used by country folk.

However, those experienced in the use of herbs did not let the practice die out. In 1864 herbalists trained in the USA founded the National Association of Medical Herbalists – now the Institute of Medical Herbalists – and they have fought to keep the use of herbs going ever since.

Now there is much medical research to back up the use of herbs for medicinal purposes and it has become very popular. When the Government recently tried to ban unlicensed herbal remedies there was huge opposition and the idea was dropped.

Although both practices use many of the same herbs, herbal medicine does differ from traditional Chinese herbalism. Unlike Western herbal medicine which has its origins in many countries, the use of Chinese herbs is deeply based in the Tao philosophy and the herbs are classified according to their properties, such as cooling, drying, damping or heating.

How the therapy works

While some drugs do have herbal origins, only the active ingredient of the plant is extracted and used. However, a herbal practitioner uses all the therapeutic parts of the plant – flowers, leaves, roots, bark, wood, berries – for treatment as they believe that it is the constituents of the plant as a whole that have medicinal effects. The herbs will be chosen depending more on the individual child at that particular time rather than the ailment they might have, so treatment works holistically on the causes rather than the symptoms of the condition.

What to expect from a first visit

The practitioner will need to build up a detailed picture of your child before deciding which herbs to prescribe. They will ask questions about your child's general health, family medical background, diet, bowel habits, sleeping patterns, as well as their type of personality. The medical herbalist's training means he or she can also carry out a physical examination, such as listening to the heart and chest, taking your child's pulse and blood pressure and examining the throat, ears and eyes. Advice may then be given on lifestyle, diet and exercise.

The herbs prescribed will suit your child for that particular time and may change at each visit. More than one will probably be given. For instance, one to help detoxify, another to help boost the immune system and another to calm the nerves. They may also be given in different forms, such as tinctures, infusions, tablets, compresses, decoctions and creams (see p.221).

The herbs taken internally can be unoffensive, but some do taste a little unpleasant. A swift gulp may work, but you may need to mix the herbs with juice.

Finding a therapist

Always ask the practitioner what experience they have of treating children as this is a specialist field and experience is advisable. Personal recommendation is also one of the best methods of finding a therapist. The following organizations will have a list of fully qualified practitioners:

The National Institute of Medical Herbalists (NIMH) 56 Longbrook Street, Exeter EX4 6AH. Tel: 01392 426022
General Council and Register of Consultant Herbalists (GCRCH) 32 King Edward's Road, Swansea SA1 4LL. Tel: 01792 655866

What qualifications to look for

Graduates of the NIMH will have trained for at least four years and, as a member, will have the initials MNIMH after their name. Fully qualified medical herbalists are trained in the same examination techniques as GPs.

Use with other therapies

Practitioners of herbal medicine may also prescribe the Bach Flower Remedies as part of their treatment. Naturopaths also use herbs as part of their treatment and it works well with most other therapies, although is probably better not used with homoeopathy to gain the best results.

Any dangers

Herbs can be extremely powerful and may be toxic if used in large doses. Their use is strictly controlled under law. But a fully qualified practitioner will prescribe what is suitable for your child and should not advise any toxic herbs. Because of this, it is much better to seek professional help from a medical herbalist rather than trying to treat your child at home. The herbal remedies available over-the-counter are also controlled and any instructions given should be followed carefully. If you are in any doubt, always consult a practitioner or doctor. If you are in any doubt about your child's symptoms, always consult your GP and always let them know if you are seeing a medical herbalist.

How much will it cost

A first consultation may cost around £18–£30 and herbs will cost extra. This can add up, depending on your child's condition and the number of visits needed. Subsequent consultations may cost around £15–£20. Herbal medicine is also covered under some private health insurance schemes.

Availability on the NHS

Although you probably won't get free treatment on the NHS, more doctors are prepared to refer patients on to clinics which may use herbal medicine.

Helpful reading

The Herb Bible Earl Mindell, Vermilion
Complete Guide to Modern Herbalism Simon Mills, Thorsons
Herbs for Common Ailments Anne McIntyre, Gaia

HOMOEOPATHY

As with so many complementary therapies, homoeopathy's origins lie with the fourth-century Greek physician Hippocrates, who believed 'like cures like'. But it was the prominent German doctor Samuel Hahnemann who, in the early 1800s, developed the method of treatment that we know today as homoeopathy by working out that substances which produce symptoms in a healthy person can cure those symptoms in a sick person.

His discovery occurred when, disillusioned with practising medicine, noting that cinchona tree bark had proved effective in treating malaria, he took a dose himself and found himself having similar symptoms – fever, headache, malaise. Every time he took a dose, the same thing happened and on this he based his 'Law of Similars'. Other doctors, drawn to his way of thinking, carried out similar experiments using animal, vegetable and mineral substances. Each remedy was 'proved', meaning all symptoms – emotional, physical, mental – were taken into account and specifically noted down. Hahnemann called his form of medicine homoeopathy, from the Greek words *omeos* meaning similar and *pathos* meaning suffering.

When using the treatments on patients, he realized that large doses could cause side-effects, so he diluted them. He carried on diluting until there was little or none of the original substance left and yet the treatment still worked. This was because by vigorously shaking or 'succussing' the solution it became more potent. The more it was diluted and succussed, the more potent it became. Homoeopaths believe that the curative power comes from the process and that 'footprints' of the original substance energize the solution.

Modern doctors still have a hard time accepting this theory. They work by fighting against disease and can't believe that such a dilute solution can possibly have a curative effect. However, it may just be that there aren't sufficiently sophisticated scientific methods for recognizing these 'footprints'. But much research has gone into homoeopathy and results are positive. So much so that as far back as 1850 the first homoeopathic hospital opened and there are now five NHS homoeopathic hospitals around the country.

How does the therapy work

Homoeopaths see illness as a sign that the inner body is out of balance. They therefore treat a patient holistically, or as a whole – taking into account their mental, physical, emotional and spiritual health – and will help the body to rebalance itself. To do this they will choose a remedy that is closest to your child's symptoms in all these areas. Of the 2000 odd remedies now available, one will be chosen that will suit every aspect of your child – whether they are outgoing or introverted, eat well or are fussy, anxious or laid back, if the symptoms are worse at a particular time or on a particular side of the body. For this reason, parents are often not told exactly which remedy is being prescribed, as although no symptoms are 'good' or 'bad', some parents may be offended by the diagnosis!

What to expect from a first visit

The first visit may last an hour or more as the homoeopath

asks detailed questions to build up an overall picture of the child. As well as more general questions about health, family medical background, diet, constitution, sleeping habits and bowel movements, the homoeopath will also ask more un-usual questions, such as on which side does your child sleep, how they react to certain weather conditions, emotional responses to situations and so on. Only once a full picture has been drawn up will a particular remedy be given. A number of pills will then be prescribed, to be taken under the tongue and as often as advised by the homoeopath (see p.224).

Finding a therapist

Always ask the practitioner what experience they have of treating children as this is a specialist field and experience is advisable. Personal recommendation is also one of the best methods of finding a therapist. There are two main organiza-tions representing homoeopaths:

The Society of Homoeopaths 2 Artizan Road, Northampton NN1 4HU. Tel: 01604 21400

British Homoeopathic Association 27a Devonshire Street, London W1N 1RJ. Tel: 0171 935 2163 (represents homoeo-paths who are also fully qualified doctors)

Further information on homoeopathy can also be obtained from:

The Hahnemann Society Hahnemann House, 2 Powis Place, Great Ormond Street, London WC1N 3HT. Tel: 0171 837 9469

What qualifications to look for

There are a wide range of training colleges, but for a profes-sional homoeopath (rather than one who is also a doctor) it is best to choose someone who has the initials RSHom after their name. This means they are a registered member of the Society, and will abide by their code of ethics and practice.

Use with other therapies

Homoeopathy can be used successfully with a number of other therapies, such as chiropractic, osteopathy and the Alexander Technique. But its use should not be combined with aromatherapy, acupuncture or herbal remedies as it may be difficult to determine which therapy is working well. If in doubt, consult your practitioner.

Any dangers

Homoeopathy is perfectly safe to use, but like with any medicine, should not be taken if your child is not ill. In fact, the remedy should be stopped as symptoms improve, and the potency never decreased during a course of treatment, otherwise the remedy may 'prove' itself and symptoms worsen. If you are in any doubt about your child's symptoms, always consult your GP. Some children may be allergic to the lactose in the little pills, but there is an alternative base available in the form of fruit sugar.

How much will it cost

A first visit may cost around £25 and subsequent visits less, depending on the type of practice you visit. The homoeopathic remedies are usually included in the price. A good rapport is essential and the homoeopath should be happy to have an initial chat without charge. Homoeopathy is now covered under many private health insurance schemes.

Availability on the NHS

Homoeopathy is widely available on the NHS and since it has been recognized by an Act of Parliament, your GP should refer you to a qualified practitioner if you ask. GPs aren't always aware of this, so they may need prompting. It may help to give them one of the numbers below. Others are still not open to the idea of homoeopathy and you may want to change GPs.

You may be referred to a clinic, a GP with homoeopathic training or one of the five homoeopathic hospitals:

The Royal London Homoeopathic Hospital NHS Trust (Tel: 0171 833 7276)

The Glasgow Homoeopathic Hospital (Tel: 0141 334 9800) and Glasgow Out-Patient Clinic for Adults and Children (Tel: 0141 771 7396/7)

Mossley Hill Hospital, Liverpool (Tel: 0151 250 3000)

United Bristol Healthcare NHS Trust (Tel: 0117 973 1231)

Kent and Sussex Weald NHS Trust Homoeopathic Hospital (Tel: 01892 542977)

Helpful reading

Miranda Castro's Guide to Mother and Baby Miranda Castro, Pan

Introductory Guide to Homoeopathy Dr Anne Clover, Thorsons

Homoeopathy Nelson Bruton, Vermilion

HYPNOTHERAPY

Hypnosis has had some bad press in recent years with the growing popularity of stage hypnotists, particularly on television. But there is a vast difference between picking out a few susceptible people from an audience and 'making' them do things and hypnotherapy.

The word hypnotherapy comes from the Greek word *hypnos*, meaning sleep. Its effects have been used down the centuries and by different civilizations, from the priests of ancient Greece to Balinese fire dancers. The Austrian doctor Franz Anton Mesmer (from whom we now have the word mesmerize) used magnets to help treat patients, although his theories were eventually discounted through lack of scientific basis. In the mid-1880s a Scottish surgeon, James Braid, used hypnosis as a method of painkilling while operating on patients. However, the technique lost favour as anaesthetics were developed. Modern hypnosis is now largely based on the methods of the American psychiatrist Dr Milton H. Erickson, who used more creative ways of helping through hypnotherapy.

Hypnosis is the tool that hypnotherapists use to enable them to help children deal with problems, by opening the subconscious mind. While the conscious mind deals only with the present, the subconscious mind stores information and only brings it to the fore when necessary. It also controls subconscious physical action such as movement and psychological functions, including emotions.

How the therapy works

The image of a hypnotherapist regressing a patient back to some trauma early on in their lives, opening the floodgates of emotion and so healing the patient, is now a largely outdated one. Many of the hypnotherapy schools see the use of regression as too aggressive and not as effective as other methods of treatment. A more popular method is to manipulate the link between an event and the negative feeling associated with it, to make good links and break bad ones. Most problems are caused by a mental link between external events (e.g. the sight of a spider) and an internal response (fear, panic). The earliest versions of hypnotherapy regressed the patient to an original trauma (a spider running across your face), but this has largely been superseded by techniques which make this sometimes traumatic regression unnecessary and instead affects the mental links themselves. For instance, a boy who has a phobia of spiders won't need to be regressed to the time he was badly scared by a spider. But he may be told to imagine himself sitting in front of the TV with the image of a cartoon spider or a man dressed up in a spider costume on the screen. As this spider is so unreal he can feel comfortable being near it. Gradually, the hypnotherapist will change the image until it seems like a real spider. The child will have broken the link that spiders are something to be afraid of and will stop associating them with fear.

Unlike stage hypnosis, your child will be safely guided into a hypnotic state. Audience participants of stage hypnosis are in fact letting themselves be carried along by suggestion and are chosen because they are extrovert and usually open to try anything.

What to expect from a first visit

The hypnotherapist will take detailed notes of your child's personal and medical history, they will also need to know of any other treatments given and any drugs administered. It may not be until the second session that your child is actually hypnotized.

The therapist should explain to your child exactly what is going to happen. They will be asked to sit or lie down and then quietly repeated suggestions that they are tired and their eyelids are becoming heavy will take them into a trance. The trance is simply a deeply relaxed state, rather like daydreaming or the feeling just before falling asleep. Your child may seem asleep, but in fact they are in a deep state of relaxation and very aware of what is being said to them. They will only reveal what they feel ready to reveal and this may be gently coaxed out in a variety of ways, such as story telling, suggestions, age regression and so on. The therapist will be observing any changes in the child as they are in the trance which will help to give clues to the root of the problem. The therapist may then teach some simple self-help hypnosis techniques which can be used at home.

Finding a therapist

Always ask the practitioner what experience they have of treating children as this is a specialist field and experience is advisable. Personal recommendation is also one of the best methods of finding a therapist. Unfortunately, the standard of training of hypnotherapists varies widely and someone who has only done a short correspondence course can call themselves a hypnotherapist. So it is important to find a therapist who has been properly trained through a recognized association rather than picking one out of the phone book. If you contact one of the following, they should send a list of fully qualified practitioners:

British Hypnosis Research (BHR) PAJE House, 164 West Wycombe Road, High Wycombe HP12 3AE. Tel: 01494 539559

Central Register of Advanced Hypnotherapists (CRAH) 28 Finsbury Park Road, London N4 2JX. Tel: 0171 359 6991

The National Register of Hypnotherapists and Psychotherapists (NRHP) 12 Cross Street, Nelson BB9 7EN. Tel: 01282 699378

UK College for Complementary Healthcare Studies St Charles Hospital, Exmoor Street, London W10 6DZ. Tel: 0181 964 1206

What qualifications to look for

Each of the above associations will have a list of therapists who have been trained at recognized colleges. Initials after their name will depend on which association they are members of, so may be MBHR, MCRAH, MNRHP and so on. Being a member of one of the above organizations means the practitioner must abide by a strict code of ethics, follow disciplinary procedures and be fully insured. Colleges offer full- or part-time training courses and the length of time spent training will reflect this.

Use with other therapies

Hypnotherapy can be used successfully with many other therapies, as it follows the similar principle that what affects the mind affects the body and vice versa. Acupuncture, reflexology, osteopathy, homoeopathy and so on may all be of benefit in conjunction with hypnosis.

Any dangers

No, not as long as you have chosen a fully qualified hypnotherapist. Ask for proof of qualifications. Depending on the problem, your child may find the sessions emotionally tiring, but with proper guidance should not become overly distressed. Check that the therapist has experience in treating children and ask to be present during the therapy.

How much will it cost

Sessions may cost from about £35 for children. Depending on the problem, only one or two sessions may be needed, but more may be necessary for deep-rooted disturbances.

Availability on the NHS

Hypnosis can be available under the NHS, but you must be referred by your doctor. Some doctors, psychiatrists and dentists use hypnosis routinely as part of their treatment.

Helpful reading

Introductory Guide to Hypnotherapy Hellmut W. A. Karle, Thorsons

KINESIOLOGY

Kinesiology (pronounced kin-easy-ology) uses gentle muscle testing to look for imbalances in the body. Then, by rubbing specific pressure points and using various kinesiology techniques, balance may be regained. Kinesiologists believe that if the muscles are in good health so is the rest of the body. When there are physical, mental or emotional upsets, the muscles become weakened and this may lead to reduced health in the future. A kinesiologist can assess the wellbeing of the whole body from testing just a few muscles.

Kinesiology, from the Greek word *kinesis*, meaning motion, is a much more modern therapy than some of its counterparts in complementary medicine. In 1965, the chiropractor Dr George Goodheart was treating a patient who had severe leg pains. He discovered that when he massaged a particular muscle, the pain eased, and that muscle had strengthened. However, massaging other muscles in the leg did nothing to help. He looked at research carried out by Dr Frank Chapman, an osteopath at the turn of the nineteenth century, and connected his findings that putting pressure on specific points improved the flow of lymph fluids through the body. He then examined the work of another osteopath, Terence Bennett, who had found that the circulation of the blood could be improved by putting light touch on certain points on the skull. By touching these points, Goodheart found that certain muscles then strengthened. In trying to work out how this was able to happen, he studied the Chinese art of acupuncture, which works on the principle that the body has invisible channels or meridians, through which energy flows, and pressure points. Acupuncturists insert needles into these points to ensure the flow of energy and so health. Goodheart adapted these findings to what is now called applied kinesiology.

How the therapy works

Kinesiologists look at the body as a whole, not just the specific symptoms set before them. They look for imbalances and weaknesses which are causing ill-health, such as a lack in nutrition or emotional upset, by putting light pressure on certain points. By gauging the strength or weakness of a muscle, a kinesiologist can tell where the weak points are. Muscle testing also assesses the body's energy meridians. Just as we have electricity that enables a light to be switched on, although we can't see the electric current, so kinesiologists work on the body's energy circuits. Ill-health, such as stress, can lead to a breakdown in these circuits and muscle testing can find where these circuits have been interrupted and restore the flow of energy and so restore health.

What to expect from a first visit

A first session may take up to an hour as the kinesiologist takes detailed notes of your child's history, from their general medical health, to any treatment given, lifestyle, diet, habits and so on. They will be asked to stand, sit or lie on a couch while different muscles are tested. The best results can be achieved by direct touch to the skin so the lymphatics can be assessed and worked on. So if your child is comfortable with this, they will be asked to undress to their vest and pants. Then they will be asked to hold out an arm or leg, for instance, and gentle pressure will be applied for a few seconds, while signs of spasm, shaking or weakening are monitored. The kinesiologist may ask for a healthy surrogate testee (probably you) if the child is too young (and restless) to be tested. If this happens, your child will be asked to touch your shoulder and the energy will be transferred through, making it easier for the kinesiologist to test.

Finding a therapist

Always ask the practitioner what experience they have of treating children as this is a specialist field and experience is advisable. Personal recommendation is also one of the best methods of finding a therapist. There are two main kinesiology organizations which can provide information on local therapists:

The Academy of Systematic Kinesiology 39 Browns Road, Surbiton KT5 8ST. Tel: 0181 399 3215

Kinesiology Federation PO Box 7891, London SW19 1ZB. Tel: 0181 545 0255

What qualifications to look for

Kinesiologists must have completed more than one hundred and fifty hours training and two hundred hours in a recognized clinic within two years.

Use with other therapies

Many other practitioners, such as chiropractors, osteopaths, naturopaths, homoeopaths and herbalists also use kinesiology as part of their treatment.

Any dangers

As there is no intrusive action and the pressure used is very light, there is no danger in using kinesiology. However, it should not be used instead of seeking medical attention, so don't put off going to see a doctor if you are worried about your child's health. Kinesiology's success can depend on the skill of the practitioner, so check on their experience first.

How much will it cost

Sessions can cost £35–£40 for children for a first session. Subsequent sessions may cost £25.

Availability on the NHS

Not used as an individual treatment within the NHS, but other therapists using treatments such as osteopathy, homoeopathy and chiropractic may incorporate it as part of their treatment.

Helpful reading

Introductory Guide to Kinesiology Anthea Courtenay and Maggie La Tournelle, Thorsons
An Introduction to Kinesiology, Brian Butler, Task Books
Kinesiology for Balanced Health, £20, Task Books (available from the Academy of Systematic Kinesiology)

NATUROPATHY

About 2500 years ago, the Greek physician Hippocrates said, 'let food be your medicine and let medicine be your food'. Therein lies the crux of naturopathy, or natural medicine, as it is also known. It is based on three basic principles: that the body has the power to heal itself, that disease and illness are a sign that the body is trying to heal itself, and that the whole person is affected by disease – body, mind and spirit – so therefore the whole person should be treated.

Naturopathy uses means to heal which down the centuries were the norm, but in the present day seem to have been forgotten as modern medicine takes over. A diet using natural ingredients and herbs, taking the waters and massage were all simple routes to a healthy life. Today, even in children, processed foods are eaten on the run, stress and busy lives mean the body is put under more and more pressure.

The modern form of naturopathy developed in the nineteenth century when Benedict Lust, a student of the Bavarian monk Father Sebastian Kneipp, took the use of hydrotherapy to the United States where it evolved into naturopathy, while in the UK it evolved under Stanley Leif. Today naturopathy encompasses a range of therapies that can help to prevent and treat many illnesses.

How the therapy works

Naturopathy helps the body to cure itself. It will use a number of means to do this, the main one being looking at the child's nutrition. It may also include herbalism, hydrotherapy, manual adjustments through osteopathy and chiropractic and exercises, fasting (although not necessarily for young children), massage and a look at lifestyle. A naturopath will look at possible causes for any ailment and treat those rather than the symptoms themselves. The end result should be the body back in perfect balance.

What to expect from a first visit

The first visit may take about an hour as the naturopath builds up a detailed picture of your child. Their eyes (iridology), tongue, nails and even hair may be looked at to determine health. Details of your child's general health, family medical history, diet, habits, bowel movements, like and dislikes will all be noted. Blood pressure and pulse may also be taken, the chest listened to and spinal joints checked.

Once the underlying cause of the illness has been identified, treatment can be given in a number of ways. This can include advice on dietary changes and mineral and vitamin supplements. Physically, osteopathy or chiropractic may be given, or another therapy such as homoeopathy or herbalism recommended.

Finding a therapist

Always ask the practitioner what experience they have of treating children as this is a specialist field and experience is advisable. Personal recommendation is also one of the best methods of finding a therapist. The General Council and Register of Naturopaths (GCRN) is the regulatory body, who will be able to tell you of a naturopath in your area. At the same address is The British College of Naturopathy and Osteopathy. The college runs special clinics for children during the week, which are free of charge.

BCNO Frazer House, 6 Netherhall Gardens, London NW3 5RR. Clinic tel: 0171 435 7830

Qualifications

Anyone can set themselves up as a naturopath, so make sure they belong to the GCRN. Belonging to this organization means they have completed a full-time four-year course at the college. Graduates should have a Naturopathic Diploma and the initials ND after their name, and/or MRN to signify they are members of the Register of Naturopaths. They may also have a BSc(Hons) in osteopathic medicine.

Use with other therapies

Naturopathy can be used successfully with many other therapies. Herbal medicine, homoeopathy, chiropractic and osteopathy may be given by the practitioner themselves or used in conjunction elsewhere. The Alexander Technique, reflexology and acupuncture can also benefit a patient.

Any dangers

There should be no dangers in naturopathic treatment so long as advice is followed sensibly, although a practitioner should not advise fasting for small children. If you are in any doubt about your child's symptoms, always consult your GP.

How much will it cost

Treatment should be around £15 for children, but quite a few sessions may be needed, depending on the child's condition.

Availability on the NHS

Dietary advice may well be given by GPs or hospitals, but the naturopathic approach of helping the body to heal itself is not widely used.

Helpful reading

Healthy by Nature Beth MacEoin, Thorsons
Better Health Through Natural Healing Ross Trattler, Thorsons
Super Foods Michael van Straten and Barbara Griggs, Dorling Kindersley

OSTEOPATHY

Osteopathy can be said to have its roots in engineering and the pioneering spirit of America in the 1800s. The man who first developed the concept that health could be related to the musculo-skeletal system – our bones, muscles, joints, ligaments and connective tissue – was Andrew Taylor Still.

Born in 1828, Still travelled with his preacher father and family, enduring the hardships faced by many pioneers at that time. He studied as an engineer and then as a physician. But when medicine couldn't save six of his own children from dying, his background made him look to structural causes for disease.

For many years he analysed skeletons and helped patients by working with the belief that illness can occur if the body's mechanical functions are weak. If muscles or ligaments are tense or go into spasm, then this can result in undue strain on other parts of the body. He believed that to help a patient, the body should be viewed as a whole – structurally, mentally and emotionally – and all should be treated together as, if one breaks down, the others are affected. By working on the body's framework, through gentle or high-velocity thrusts, and using massage and manipulation, the structure can return to normal as can health.

Although he had many grateful patients, others accused him of being a grave-snatcher and of being possessed. But in 1892 he opened the American School of Osteopathy. The medical establishment tried to dismiss Still and the School, but legal status was eventually obtained and osteopathy has been an integral part of US medical practice for many years. More recently, it has gained legal status in the UK, too, and is now fully available within the NHS.

How the therapy works

Osteopathy uses massage, manipulation and stretching techniques to help rebalance the musculo-skeletal system. When our muscles become tense, for instance, after a fall or due to stress, they burn up a lot of wasted energy and can be easily damaged. This tenseness slows down the circulation and can restrict breathing as well as the elimination process. This particularly refers to the joints of the spine. As the spine protects the spinal cord which makes up the major part of the nervous system, controlling voluntary and involuntary movement, re-adjusting these joints can bring relief to every other single part of the body. This may be done with soft manipulation to tissue, or the use of rhythmic movements or even high-velocity thrusts to joints, which although they look painful, should not hurt at all.

Some osteopaths will specialize in certain areas, such as cranial techniques, where the bones of the skull are very gently manipulated and moved into place. Cranial osteopathy, a more subtle form of treatment, works particularly well on babies and small children, whose bones are more easily adjusted and may have been affected during a difficult birth.

What to expect from a first visit

A first visit will probably last about an hour as the osteopath will want to build up a clear picture of your child and their health. This will include questions about any medical treatment and whether they have had any operations. They will also want to know about family background, eating habits, physical, mental and emotional wellbeing. Your child will probably be asked to strip down to their underwear and do a few simple movements so that their posture, spine alignment and mobility can be analysed and any weaknesses identified. At this stage, the osteopath may decide that this type of treatment will not be able to help your child and may refer on to another type of practitioner.

If treatment is advised, your child will be asked to lie on a table. First, gentle massage will help to relax the muscles and then rhythmic movements and stretching exercises will be done to help improve mobility. The high velocity thrusts, which can help free up joints are not usually used on children. Your child may feel very sleepy after sessions as the body relaxes.

Finding a therapist

Since the passing of the 1993 Osteopaths Act, osteopathy is now state regulated, meaning that legally osteopaths are as professional as doctors or dentists. Your GP can refer you to a fully qualified osteopath, or The Osteopathic Information Service has a list of osteopaths currently registered:

Osteopathic Information Service (OIS) PO Box 2074, Reading RG1 4YR. Tel: 01734 512051

Osteopathic Centre for Children (OCC) 19a Cavendish Square, Harcourt House, London W1M 9AD. Tel: 0171 495 1231. The OCC has clinics Monday to Friday and on Saturday mornings (a donation of £15 is suggested, but fees are flexible). A satellite clinic has recently opened in Dublin.

The British College of Naturopathy and Osteopathy (BCNO) Frazer House, 6 Netherhall Gardens, London NW3 5RR. Tel: 0171 435 7830. The BCNO holds a children's clinic Monday to Friday (free to children under 16).

What qualifications to look for

Only those who have registered with the newly set up General Osteopathic Council can legally practise as osteopaths. Members must have undertaken a four-year full-time course or six years part-time and should have the letters DO, MRO after their name. Training covers subjects such as anatomy, pathology, biomechanics, physiology, sociology and psychology. Practitioners must follow a code of practice and of ethics and be fully insured. Always ask the practitioner what experience they have of treating children as this is a specialist field and experience is advisable. Personal recommendation is also one of the best methods of finding a therapist.

Use with other therapies

Osteopathy works very well with some therapies such as herbal medicine, naturopathy and homoeopathy. Some of the other therapies, such as chiropractic, acupuncture and reflexology, might be avoided until osteopathic treatment is finished, but check with your practitioner.

Any dangers

There are some conditions for which osteopathy is not suitable, so it is always advisable to give a practitioner as many details about your child's general health as possible. Osteopathy should not hurt and the gentler actions work very well for children.

How much will it cost

Treatment costs around £25, depending on the individual practitioner. Osteopathy is covered under many private health insurance schemes.

Availability on the NHS

Osteopathy is widely used within the NHS. Many doctors are very happy to refer you to a qualified practitioner or may have one within the surgery. Osteopathy is also generally used in hospitals to help with a variety of conditions. Many, if not all, private healthcare insurance companies are also happy to cover payment for osteopathy.

Helpful reading

Introductory Guide to Osteopathy Edward D. O. Triance, Thorsons
Osteopathy, Stephen Sandler, Vermilion

REFLEXOLOGY

Reflexology has been used for many thousands of years. A wall painting, dating from 2000 years BC, found in a physician's tomb at Saqqara in Egypt shows men applying pressure to the feet of others. It has been used by many other cultures, too – native American Indian tribes, the Chinese and Africans.

But it wasn't until the early part of the twentieth century that a more modern form came into common use. An American ear, nose and throat specialist, Dr William Fitzgerald, devised a system which applied pressure through the hands to certain parts of the body, known as zone therapy. A student of his work, physiotherapist Eunice Ingham took his work further by saying that the different areas of the body could be treated by working on the feet which she felt were more sensitive; and it was one of her students, Doreen Bayley, who brought this form of reflexology to the UK in the 1960s.

Reflexology is based on the belief that each part of the body is connected by energy pathways which all end in the feet and hands. There are ten vertical zones, five on each side of the body, which run from the head, down the arms and to the toes and all the body parts within each zone are linked by the energy pathways (see illustration). An organ within a particular zone will have a reflex site within the same zone on the foot. But illness, stress, bad diet and emotional upset can all block the energy pathways. By working on the zone in the foot, the energy block can be freed and health returned.

These reflex points are also found on the hands, but it is thought the feet are more sensitive to touch and are larger, making treatment easier (see drawing opposite).

REGIONS OF THE FOOT USED IN REFLEXOLOGY

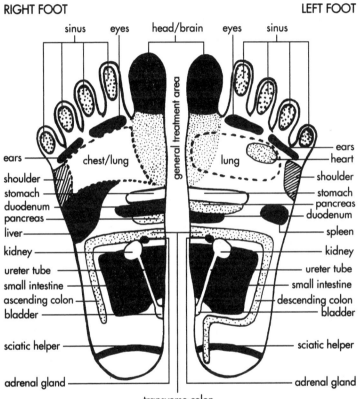

RIGHT FOOT

LEFT FOOT

sinus · eyes · head/brain · eyes · sinus

general treatment area

ears
chest/lung · lung
shoulder
stomach
duodenum
pancreas
liver
kidney
ureter tube
small intestine
ascending colon
bladder

sciatic helper

adrenal gland

ears
heart
shoulder
stomach
pancreas
duodenum
spleen
kidney
ureter tube
small intestine
descending colon
bladder

sciatic helper

adrenal gland

transverse colon

How the therapy works

As reflexologists treat the person holistically – as a whole – the entire foot will be worked on. Gentle manipulation, using massage and pressure on the reflex points, will not only help the problem by releasing blockages but will be relaxing for the child. Tenderness in some areas will show where the problem may lie. Some complaints may clear up after just one or two sessions, while others may take longer.

What to expect from a first visit

A first session may last about an hour as the reflexologist asks questions about your child's health, background, diet, personality and lifestyle. They will also need to know if your child is on any medication and has had any operations. Your child will then be asked to lie on a couch and their feet will be examined. The reflexologist will analyse the skin, colour, temperature and tissue of the feet as well as look for signs of infection. Reflexology does not tickle, although your child may feel discomfort or even pain in the area where there is a blockage, but the pressure will be adjusted to suit them. And as the treatment progresses, these areas should become less sensitive. As a sign that the body is going through the healing process, some symptoms may get worse before they get better. Many people tend to feel very tired after a session and your child may want to sleep.

Finding a therapist

Always ask the practitioner what experience they have of treating children as this is a specialist field and experience is advisable. Personal recommendation is also one of the best

methods of finding a therapist. There are a number of reflexology organizations. The British Complementary Medicine Association will send a list of member organizations.
BCMA, 9 Soar Lane, Leicester LE3 5DE. Tel: 0116 242 5406
Association of Reflexologists 27 Old Gloucester Street, London WC1N 3XX. Tel: 01935 817617. Has over 1200 members.

What qualifications to look for

There are many organizations which belong to the BCMA, such as the International Federation of Reflexologists, The British Reflexology Association, the Association of Reflexologists and so on. Each may offer full- or part-time courses and qualifications will depend on this. When contacting each organization, ask which qualifications they expect their members to have.

Use with other therapies

Reflexology can be used with a number of other therapies, such as osteopathy, acupuncture and chiropractic. It may be best to avoid using it in conjunction with aromatherapy, herbal medicine and homoeopathy, as it may be difficult to tell which therapy is working well.

Any dangers

Although giving your child a gentle foot rub will always benefit them if they are feeling under the weather, a trained reflexologist can 'reach' parts you cannot and will know when extra care is needed or whether special attention is called for if medication is being used. If epilepsy runs in the family, or your child is diabetic, reflexology should be avoided.

How much will it cost

A first session may cost around £16 for a child, although subsequent sessions may be less, about £10. Reflexology is covered under some private health insurance schemes.

Availability on the NHS

It is not common to be referred on for reflexology by GPs, although some do practise it themselves. Reflexology is available in some NHS hospitals, but it depends on their individual policy.

Helpful reading

Introductory Guide to Reflexology, Nicola M. Hall, Thorsons
Reflexology for Children Kevin and Barbara Kunz, Thorsons
Reflexology Anya Gore, Vermilion

TRADITIONAL CHINESE MEDICINE (TCM)

Traditional Chinese medicine has been used for many thousands of years in the prevention and treatment of illness. The first words written about this form of medicine, the *Nei Ching*, were written down in AD 400 and known as the Yellow Emperor's Classics of Internal Medicine. TCM is not one but many therapies, and can include Chinese herbs, acupuncture, massage, moxibustion, diet and movement, such as t'ai chi. Herbal medicine, acupuncture, moxibustion and other therapies often viewed as being 'traditionally Chinese' are also a part of the traditions of Japan, Korea and Tibet. While TCM has come to be the best known of these traditions, all are branches of Oriental medicine as a whole.

Chinese medicine has to be looked at from a totally different standpoint to Western medicine. While conventional doctors will treat the symptoms, only sometimes looking for causes, a practitioner of Chinese medicine will see the symptoms only as a sign of something deeper. TCM treats the patient as a whole – that the mental, physical and emotional are all linked – and will try to diagnose causes and treat them so eventually the symptoms may disappear.

The philosophy behind TCM is that good health depends on the flow around the body of Qi (pronounced chee) or vital energy. This energy moves through invisible channels or meridians. There are fourteen meridians, seven *yin* and seven *yang*. Yin and yang are opposing, yet complementary forces. Yin is seen as the dark, feminine, cold force and represents the dense, blood-filled organs such as the liver and heart. Yang is seen as the light, male, warm side and represents the organs concerned with discharge and digestion such as the bladder and stomach. We are also further considered to be made up of five elements – wood, fire, earth, metal and water.

When in perfect health, the two forces are in perfect balance. But if one dominates and there is an excess of yin or yang, then ill health or disease can develop. The Chinese believe there can be many causes leading to this. There are the external energies of dampness, wind, dryness, cold, heat and summer heat, or the emotions or bad diet and fatigue may play a part. For instance, if there is too much fire in the body, then the skin may become inflamed, if there is too much damp, then phlegm can result. These can all affect the flow of Qi through the body and the practitioner of Chinese medicine will use various methods to free the flow of energy and restore balance.

How the therapy works

Children will be diagnosed differently to adults, especially infants. TCM practitioners believe that 90 per cent of ailments in the under threes are digestive or respiratory in origin and special attention will be paid to these areas.

The Chinese have built up a list of therapeutic herbs over thousands of year and each will be chosen for their effect on particular organs. So a 'cold' herb may be used if there is an excess of heat in the body. Unlike homoeopathy, where only one remedy is given, a mixture of herbs will be prepared.

Heating the pressure points, known as moxibustion, may also be used. Small amounts of the herb moxa is burnt in a cone and either held over a pressure point or stuck on a needle to help stimulate the point. Diet, lifestyle and exercise will also be looked at and may be included in treatment.

Acupuncture is also commonly used in TCM (see also p.150) as well as Chinese herbs. If acupuncture is used, needles will be inserted on some of the 365 main pressure points along the meridians during treatment which will help to free the flow of vital energy.

What to expect from a first visit

The practitioner of Chinese medicine will want to build up a detailed picture of your child before making a diagnosis. Questions about their general health, lifestyle, habits, personality, likes and dislikes, how they fit into the family, sleep routines, bowel habits, emotions and so on will be asked. Your child's tongue will be examined as the Chinese believe the condition of the tongue – its texture, coating, colour and shape – are all significant. Your child's pulse will also be taken – the practitioner will feel for six on each wrist, which correspond to different organs, although in younger children, the pulse will only be in one place on each wrist, or on the neck and ankles. Only then will the practitioner decide which type of treatment will best suit your child (see p.227).

Finding a therapist

At present anyone can set up as a practitioner in Chinese herbal medicine but all reputable practitioners trained in Chinese herbs in this country are members of the Register of Chinese Herbal Medicine. Be sure to find a practitioner through one of the recognized organizations (below). Always ask the practitioner what experience they have of treating children as this is a specialist field and experience is advisable. If you can, reinforce your choice of practitioner through personal recommendation. (See also under Acupuncture.)
Register of Chinese Herbal Medicine PO Box 400, Wembley HA6 9NZ. Tel: 0181 908 1697
British Acupuncture Council Park House, 206–208 Latimer Road, London W10 6RE. Tel: 0181 964 0222

What qualifications to look for

Even if a practitioner claims to have trained in China this does not mean they are experienced in prescribing what can be very toxic herbs. Only use a practitioner who is fully qualified and is a member of one of the above organizations. A practitioner should have the initials MRCHM (member of the Register of Chinese Herbal Medicine) after their name. If your child is under seven, ask if they have done a specialist paediatric training, as in TCM children are treated as a separate discipline. They should have had training in herbs for a minimum of four years (i.e. three years TCM, one year paediatrics).

Use with other therapies

Acupuncture and Chinese herbal medicine are often used in tandem. Other therapies such as homoeopathy and medical herbalism and any other orally taken remedies should be avoided until you are certain whether the treatment is working or not.

Any dangers

The herbs prescribed should be suited to your child if given by a fully qualified practitioner, as a few are toxic. Experimenting with herbs or using a practitioner who cannot prove they have recognized training in this country should be avoided. Some herbal practitioners now monitor liver function with blood tests to prevent any risk of liver toxicity from certain herbs.

How much will it cost

A first session will cost about £20–£45, and subsequent sessions from £15 upwards, depending on where you live.

Availability on the NHS

Traditional Chinese medicine is available on the NHS, but you are more likely to be treated if referred to a hospital or associated clinic. For instance, at Great Ormond Street Hospital for Sick Children in London the dermatology department may refer on to a Chinese doctor who acts as a research consultant, and many children have benefited when conventional treatment has failed them.

Helpful reading

Chinese Herbal Medicine Dr Guang Xu, Vermilion

OTHER THERAPIES

The following therapies can also be beneficial in treating some of the ailments included in the A–Z section. Fact-finding for this book has found research studies supporting the benefits of some of the therapies, for instance yoga in the treatment of asthma. However, enquiries found them not to be used as much for children as are the therapies in the main part of this section. Remember to always ask the practitioner what experience they have of treating children, as this is a specialist field.

Alexander Technique

The Alexander Technique is a system of re-learning how to use posture, balance and movement in every day life. If we use our bodies properly, so that the head freely balances on the top of the spine, then the muscular and skeletal systems are aligned and work efficiently. Although children are less likely to suffer problems such as bad posture, backache and impaired movement, modern schools with plastic chairs and flat desks do nothing to help prevent such problems arising. Stress, injury and emotional upset can all lead to neck and back problems as the body tenses up, causing the spine to shorten. An Alexander teacher will help a child to learn – or re-learn – how to use themselves properly again. What will start out as conscious movements, such as standing up without craning the head forward, will eventually become an unconscious act through repetitive teaching.

Stress, asthma, backache and other problems can be alleviated through using the Alexander Technique. Around
twenty-five sessions are usually needed, costing about
£12–£25 each. It is not generally available on the NHS,
although some schools have invited teachers to show pupils
how it can work.

Society of Teachers of the Alexander Technique (STAT) 20
London House, 266 Fulham Road, London SW10 9EL. Tel:
0171 351 0828

Colour Therapy

We use terms such as 'seeing red' or being 'green with envy' or
'feeling blue'. We also describe people's health through colour
– they may look pale, rosy or green – which all reflects its
importance on our lives. A grey day can make all the difference
between feeling happy and energetic or lethargic and there is
psychological research to back up the effect colour has on us.

The sun gives out electromagnetic wavelengths, some of
which we see as natural light. The light is made up of prisms
of colour – red, yellow, orange, green, blue, turquoise, vio-
let and magenta. Other wavelengths are invisible, such as
infrared and ultraviolet light. Colour therapists believe that
the body absorbs these colours and emits its own, in the form
of an aura. When we are healthy, these colours are in balance,
but when ill, some may dominate while others may be lacking. Various methods of colour testing will be done to find
out which these are and to redress the balance through light
treatment or the use of pigment.

The Institute of Complementary Medicine PO Box 194, London
SE16 1QZ. Tel: 0171 237 5165 (10am–12.30pm) has a list of
colour therapists.

Iridology

Iridologists believe that by studying the iris of the eye, physical and mental health can be analysed. Its brightness, colour, speckling, marks and clarity are all tell-tale signs of not only your present condition but of future problems and past health. Iridologists see the iris as a map, representing different parts of the body and will use a magnifier and torch to help make their diagnosis. For instance, the left eye represents the left side of the body. A dark ring around the iris means that there is a difficulty in eliminating waste, while white specks can point to a problem in the nervous system. It is also thought that people with different coloured eyes are more prone to different problems. Those with blue or grey eyes have a tendency to produce mucus and so are more inclined to have asthma while those with brown eyes are more inclined to problems with the blood, such as anaemia.

Iridology is only used as a diagnostic tool and isn't a treatment in itself. Homoeopaths, naturopaths, aromatherapists and herbalists may use it as part of diagnosis before deciding on treatment. Although a practitioner may take a brief look at the iris of a child under six years old, full diagnosis cannot be made as the iris does not form properly until after this age. *Guild of Naturopathic Iridologists* 94 Grosvenor Road, London SW1V 3LF. Tel: 0171 834 3579

Massage

Massage is second nature to us all, including children. We rub an injury better, we massage our temples during a headache, or our eyes when tired. It is a practice of hands on the body that is thousands of years old, but its real therapeutic effects have gone in and out of fashion down the centuries. It is now very popular as it is easy to practise and can bring light relief in a short period of time.

There are many different forms of massage, such as remedial, manual lymphatic drainage, shiatsu, rolfing, physiotherapy and so on. Light massage can stimulate the nerve endings in the skin, causing the body to relax. Deeper massage can work on specific areas to stimulate the circulation and eliminate toxins or knead tightened muscles and tissue. Massage is used widely in NHS hospitals and also in some GP surgeries. Many nurses are now trained in its use and it is incorporated as part of treatment from newborn babies to children with constipation and broken legs.

Massage sessions usually last at least three quarters of an hour and cost from about £15.

British Massage Therapy Council Greenbank House, 65a Adelphi Street, Preston PR1 7BH. Tel: 01772 881063

Nutritional Therapy

Nutritional therapists believe that all disease is influenced in some way by nutrition and that with an appropriate diet problems such as migraine, skin eruptions and lack of resistance to infection can be treated. There are three main criteria a therapist will look at in a child before deciding on the best diet. The first is identifying any food or environmental intolerances or allergies. The second is to detect any toxic overload in the system, a poor ability to eliminate waste or poor liver function. And the third is to look for nutritional deficiencies due to a poor diet and whether the patient has any problems with malabsorption or any special needs. Diagnosis will be made through questioning and examination, and also via laboratory testing of blood, urine, sweat and hair. Costs can vary between £20 and £40 for

an hour's session, plus extra for any products recommended.

The Society for the Promotion of Nutritional Therapy, PO Box 47,
Heathfield TN21 8ZX. Tel: 01435 867007. Members of the
Society include doctors, nurses and clinical scientists as well as
complementary therapists.

Sound Therapy

We are often oblivious to sounds around us until one particular one strikes a chord and effects us in some way. The sound
of a car horn can jangle on the nerves, the rousing football
song can excite a whole spectator audience, the song of a bird
can make you feel happy, repeating a mantra can bring tran-
quillity. In modern medicine, hospitals use high intensity
sound to disintegrate gall stones while ultrasound is used to
scan the form of an unborn baby in the womb.

Sound therapists believe that, when healthy, parts of the
body have a natural resonance or frequency. When that resonance is affected, then so is health. Our whole body actually
absorbs sound and therapists say that by directing sound at different parts of the body, some conditions can be alleviated
and the resonance restored. Also, by learning how to use your
voice properly and creating different sounds, physical, mental
and emotional health can all be positively affected. Sound is
also used as part of music and dance therapy which can be
practised at home. The use of sound and voices to help heal
is not greatly recognized in the NHS, unless high-tech equip-
ment is used. Sessions or workshops can cost from about £15.

There is not an overall sound therapy organization in this
country. But sound healer Susan Lever runs nationwide
workshops and sessions and can be contacted about local
therapists. Send an sae to:

Susan Lever 2 Woodlea, Coulby Newham, Middlesborough TS8 0TX. Tel: 01642 590562

Yoga

Yoga combines spiritual, mental and physical training and can help a range of ailments from asthma to muscular injuries and stress-related problems such as sleeping difficulties. The most common form of yoga is known as *hatha* yoga and it works through posture or *asanas* and breathing exercises or *pranayama*. The yoga philosophy emphasizes the influence of mind over body.

The yoga exercises are carried out slowly and methodically with breathing and often incorporate visualization. In yoga, breathing is seen as the child's (or adult's) life force or *prana*. Controlled breathing can help bring relaxation, while the postures help muscle tension. This makes yoga beneficial for problems such as asthma and other respiratory problems, stress and backache. Studies have shown that doing yoga exercises can improve the breathing of asthmatics, causing an improvement in expiratory flow rates and leading to a reduction in the amount of drugs required.

Yoga is usually taught on a group basis, although private tuition is available. Payment is up to the individual teacher. Classes cost about £2–£5. Yoga is not generally available on the NHS, although some hospitals may include breathing techniques as part of their treatment.

The British Wheel of Yoga 1 Hamilton Place, Boston Road, Sleaford, Lincolnshire NG34 7ES. Tel: 01529 306851

The Yoga Biomedical Trust, PO Box 140, Cambridge CB4 3SY

OTHER HELPFUL ORGANIZATIONS

• *Action Against Allergy* 24–26 High Street, Hampton Hill TW12 1PD

Offers advice and a range of books on allergy and intolerance.

• *Cry-Sis* BMCry-Sis London WC1N 3XX. Tel: 0171 404 5011

Help and information for parents with babies who cry persistently.

• *Hyperactive Children's Support Group* 71 Whyke Lane, Chichester PO19 2LD. Tel: 01903 725182 (Tue–Fri, 10am–1pm)

Network of local groups offering support.

• *The Informed Parent* 19 Woodlands Road, Harrow HA1 2RT. Tel: 0181 861 1022

Provides support and information on vaccinations. It does not recommend or advise against vaccination, but helps parents to be better informed before making a decision.

• *The JABS Group (Justice, Awareness and Basic Support)* Tel: 01942 713565/01204 796433

Provides information on vaccinations and tries to help parents who believe their children may have been harmed by immunization.

• *Meningitis Research* Old Gloucester Road, Alveston, Bristol BS12 2LQ. Tel: 01454 281811; 24-hour helpline: 01454 413344

Help and information on meningitis.

• *National Asthma Campaign* Providence House, Providence Place, London N1 0NT. Tel: 0171 226 2260

Information and advice on asthma.

• *National Eczema Society* 4 Tavistock Place, London WC1H 9RA. Tel: 0171 388 4097

Information and advice on eczema.

• *The National Society for Research into Allergy* PO Box 45, Hinckley LE10 1JY. Tel: 01455 851546

Advice on allergies as well as information on alternative food sources.

• *Parentline* Tel: 01702 559900

Confidential helpline for parents concerned about any sort of problem with their children.

• *The Soil Association* 86 Colston Street, Bristol BS1 5BB. Tel: 0117 9290661

Information on national organic producers and suppliers.

• *What Doctors Don't Tell You/The Centre for Truth in Medicine* 4 Wallace Road, London N1 2PG. Tel: 0171 354 4592

SECTION III

Remedies for the Home

There are many complementary remedies that can be used safely in the home although it is always better to consult a practitioner initially when looking after the health of your child. Once you have an understanding of complementary remedies, then they can be used for acute problems and for minor complaints in the home.

Complementary therapies should not be used as an alternative to conventional medicine without first consulting your practitioner or doctor. If you are in any doubt as to your child's wellbeing you should seek medical advice first.

Aromatherapy

Essential oils are wonderful to have in the home and can be used in a number of ways to help children:

Steam inhalation One or two drops of oil are added to a bowl of boiling water. A towel is placed over the head of the child as they lean over the bowl to keep in the steam. This is one of the quickest ways for a child to feel the benefits of the oils as the inhalation sends messages to the brain and enters the bloodstream via the lungs. Children with asthma should avoid this method. *Vaporizers* There are electric vaporizers which let the aroma of the oils waft around the room and can be bought in most department stores. There are also dispensers which have a bowl for water at the top and an opening for a candle underneath. Four drops of oil are added and, once lit, the candle warms and diffuses the oils around the room, allowing a gentle method of inhalation. However, children shouldn't be left alone with these because of the risk of fire.

Handkerchief/pillow One or two drops of an essential oil on a handkerchief to inhale and/or on a pillow slip at night can help congestion and breathing difficulties as well as aid sleep.

Massage Oils for massage should never be used directly, but always diluted in a carrier oil, such as olive, almond, grapeseed or sunflower. If you intend to use massage regularly, it makes sense to make up a 50ml bottle and store it ready for use. Eight drops of oil in 50ml of carrier oil and shaken well is suitable for children aged one to twelve. For children under one, five drops of oil in 50ml of carrier oil is recommended.

Baths One to three drops of essential oil added to your child's bath will not only help to relieve any aches or pains, but the smell should arouse their interest. Always thoroughly swish the oils in the bath to mix properly before the child gets in. Use the more gentle oils, such as Lavender, in case of skin irritation. Foot (or hand) baths are also useful for problems such as fungal infections, blisters and verrucae.

Compress A compress can be made by seeping a cotton cloth in a small bowl of hand-hot water to which two or three drops of essential oils have been well mixed. Lightly squeeze out the cloth and apply to the affected area, such as a headache, bruise or swelling. Alternate hot and cold compresses can be given.

Mouth wash If your child is old enough not to swallow the wash (check with plain water first) then these can be very effective for throat infections, ulcers and toothache. Add four drops of essential oils to a cup of water (preferably distilled) and give to gargle. If a small amount is swallowed by accident, it should do no harm.

Aromatherapy first aid

Chamomile Roman Can help a range of ailments, from skin problems such as itchiness or nappy rash, to indigestion, teething and wounds.

Eucalyptus Helpful for breathing problems associated with catarrh, asthma and bronchitis. Also for digestive and circulatory conditions. (It is thought *Eucalyptus smithii* is more suitable for young children than *Eucalyptus globulus*.

Lavender Its antiseptic qualities make it useful for acne, blisters and cold sores as well as helping problems such as thrush, headaches and sprains.

Tea-Tree Useful for viral, bacterial and fungal infections, such as sore throats, colds, athlete's foot. Also good as an antiseptic for cuts and grazes.

Aromatherapy is not meant as an alternative to conventional medicine, but can help complement your child's treatment. If you are in any doubt about your child's health, consult your GP or aromatherapist.

No essential oils should be taken internally as they are very powerful. They should always be diluted in a carrier oil unless otherwise directed, for instance, a small dab of Lavender or Tea-Tree oil can occasionally be dabbed directly on a minor cut or sting. Avoid the eye, nose, mouth and genital area when using oils.

Keep your oils away from sunlight, in a dark container or bottle which has a dropper, allowing only a drop at a time to come out. If properly kept, the oils should last for about six months. Always keep the oils out of the reach of children.

Bach Flower Remedies

The Bach Flower Remedies are one of the few complementary options suggested in this book which can be recommended for initial use at home rather than first seeking the advice of a qualified practitioner. Many complementary therapists, such as herbalists, reflexologists and acupuncturists will use Bach Flower Remedies as part of their complete treatment.

The thirty-eight Bach Flower Remedies are harmless remedies which can be given to children. Not only are non-poisonous plants used, but none of the plant is actually ingested, rather it is the energy from a plant that heals by affecting the mind and emotions and so the child's wellbeing, not the plant itself.

The only other ingredient added to the remedy is brandy, which acts as a preservative. Although this may seem worrying, once the remedies have been diluted before administering (see below), the amount of brandy drunk by the child is minute, so should not be a cause for concern. The remedies come in a concentrated form known as a stock remedy. Water is then added, as below, for use. The stock remedy should be kept in a cool, dark place and can last indefinitely. Once diluted, the remedy can last up to three weeks, if kept in the fridge.

Using the Remedies

Up to six or seven remedies can be used together at the same time.

Two drops of each remedy should be added to a 30ml bottle containing natural, non-gas spring water. From the bottle, four drops should be taken, four times a day, but especially first thing in the morning and last thing at night.

The 30ml bottles can be bought from most large

chemists. The remedies can be given directly, or added to water, juice or even food. For breastfeeding babies, the diluted remedy can be dabbed on the nipple before feeding, or if the mother takes the remedy herself, the effect will filter through to her baby. If you prefer your baby not to take the remedy internally, it can be dabbed on to the temples, fontanelle, wrists and beneath the ears.

Ideally, the remedy should be given at four well-spaced times during the day. Obviously, if your child is at nursery or school, this can prove difficult, so one can be given in the morning and the other three at intervals during the afternoon and evening when they're back home. Sterilize bottles once the dilution is finished by boiling in water, before adding more.

Rescue Remedy

Rescue Remedy is particularly useful to have at home as it works well for many minor emergencies, from grazed knees and bruises to shock after falling. It is the combination of five remedies – Cherry Plum, Clematis, Impatiens, Rock Rose and Star of Bethlehem. It comes in a liquid and cream form, the latter of which also contains the cleansing remedy, Crab Apple. The liquid form should be used as follows: four drops of Rescue Remedy added to a glass of water and sipped until relief is obtained.

None of the remedies is meant as a substitute for medical care. If you are worried about your child's ailment, seek medical attention.

Herbal Medicine

As with any of the complementary therapies, where a remedy is to be taken internally it is always preferable to seek the advice of a fully qualified practitioner. A practitioner is trained to use and prescribe herbs that will suit your child individually and these will not necessarily be the same herbs that you would buy over the counter. As a practitioner will analyse the causes of any illness before prescribing, any herbs listed under herbal medicine in the A–Z of this book are included as a guide to what may be recommended and are not meant as a suggestion of what to buy.

Buying herbal medicines

Many herbs have restricted use and can be dangerous if not administered under strict guidance. However, many of the well-known brands available in this country are perfectly safe to use and can be prescribed by a doctor under the NHS. But there are other products available that claim medicinal powers and are usually sold under the guise of food. Always buy herbs from your practitioner or a reputable brand. The labelling of over-the-counter products should identify what the medicine is to be used for and give information on dosage and suitability for children or for use during pregnancy and breastfeeding.

Usage

There are different ways in which herbal medicine can be taken. Your child's herbalist will choose the one they feel is most suited to the presenting condition. Always follow closely any advice given by the practitioner on the use of the herbs.

A practitioner may advise one of the following when taking herbs:

Tincture This is the most popular form of prescribing herbs. They may be made up for you or can be made at home. Put 4oz (110g) of chopped-up herbs in a container, add one pint (520ml) of alcohol, such as vodka or gin, and seal. Leave for two weeks in a warm, dry place and shake twice a day. Then pour the liquid into a dark bottle, straining out the herbs. Seal and use when needed. Always check tincture dosages with your practitioner or use a reputable herbal medicine book.

Infusion Fresh or dried herbs are made from the soft parts of plants, such as the flower or leaf and are brewed like a tea which can then be drunk or gargled. Warm a teapot and add one teaspoon (5ml) of the herb(s) per cup of boiling water. Let the brew infuse for ten to fifteen minutes and then cool before drinking. For children under twelve, half a cup (110ml) should be taken three times a day. For babies under six months, one teaspoon (5ml) three times a day.

Decoction This uses the hard part of the plant, such as the bark. Add one heaped teaspoon (5ml) of herbs to one pint (520ml) of boiling water and bring to the boil again in a saucepan (not aluminium). Simmer for ten to fifteen minutes and then immediately strain and leave to cool before drinking. For children under twelve, half a cup (110ml) should be taken three times a day. For babies under six months, one teaspoon (5ml) three times a day.

Tisane These are similar to infusions, but come in teabags, and do not need to be brewed for as long.

Poultice Fresh herbal leaves can be applied directly to the affected area, such as a cut or graze and held in place by gauze. Or the herbs can be chopped and mixed with hot water to make a paste and then applied.

Compress These can be made by soaking a clean cloth or cotton wool in a decoction or infusion and held against the affected area.

Ointment/cream These can be given by the herbalist or can be bought over the counter from health shops.

Herbal first aid

Aloe Vera Works particularly well for burns and scalds.
Chamomile Good for stomach upsets and diarrhoea, also has a calming effect, so helpful when children are anxious or finding it difficult to sleep.
Elderflower Helpful for fever and catarrh as it will draw out the symptoms and help to cool.
Nettle Useful to apply to skin conditions such as eczema.
Lemon Balm Helps aid relaxation, but also good for the digestive system.
Peppermint Useful for the early stages of a cold for nasal decongestion. Also helps with nausea, for instance during travelling.

Homoeopathy

There are about 2000 different remedies a homoeopath can choose from. Each one is totally individual and will be given in a particular set of circumstances, depending on your child's health, background, habits, feelings and so on. This is why it is important to visit a trained homoeopath who can decide which remedy may be able to help treat your child.

The homoeopathic remedies listed under some of the ailments in the A–Z section of this book may well be recommended when you go for consultation, but they are included merely as a guide to what you might be given. They are not meant as a suggestion if you decide to buy remedies over the counter, as only with the training a homoeopath has, is it possible to look at all underlying causes of any illness – physical, emotional and mental – and decide which is the best remedy for your child. Shop-bought remedies can be helpful, but seeking the advice of a qualified, experienced homoeopath is always preferable when first starting treatment. Once you feel you have a fuller knowledge of the remedies then buying becomes easier.

This is particularly important when treating chronic conditions such as asthma, hayfever, bronchiolitis and so on. Such conditions can deteriorate and should always be monitored under qualified supervision, not just treated at home. But the more minor or acute ailments, such as colds, teething, thrush and so on can be easily and safely treated. There is, for instance, an effective homoeopathic ointment for burns (which contains Calendula, Urtica Urens, Echinacea, Hypericum and Cantharsis) available from Nelsons (see p.164), which can prevent blistering and scarring if applied rapidly.

It is worth knowing, for the future, how to use the remedies and their potencies.

Dosage

- One remedy is taken at a time and one tablet is one dose.
- For a very serious complaint, such as a bad fall, one dose should be taken every five to fifteen minutes.
- For a serious complaint, such as a sore throat, one dose should be taken every one to two hours.
- For a less serious complaint, such as the beginnings of a cold, one dose should be taken every four to eight hours.

As the symptoms change, so the dosage can be changed. Stop

giving the tablets once there is a definite improvement. If there is no sign of improvement after about six doses, then stop the treatment as it is not working and you may want to try something else, or ask for advice from your homoeopath or GP.

Usage

Put the pill under your child's tongue, where it will quickly dissolve. Try not to let your child eat or brush their teeth for about fifteen minutes before and after taking the pill. The remedies should be kept in a cool, dark place and away from any strong-smelling products such as perfume or cleaning fluids. Tea, coffee and mint should be avoided.

Potencies

The remedies are made from mineral, plant and animal substances. The prepared substance is then diluted and succussed. Succussion involves hitting the vial against a solid object. The remedies are then made up in a lactose or fruit sugar bases. It is the succussing that is said to 'potentize' the solution, giving it its powers, and the more it is diluted and succussed, the more powerful it becomes.

There are two scales of dilution and remedies are known by how much they are diluted and shaken:

- the decimal (x potency): one part of tincture to nine parts alcohol is known as 1x and so on
- centesimal (C potency): one part tincture to 999 parts alcohol and diluted and shaken twice more is known as 3C and so on.

The most commonly sold over-the-counter potency is 6C.

Once the condition begins to improve, reduce the medication or stop.

Homoeopathic first aid

Aconite For the early stages of a cold or if the child has caught a chill, if the child is upset, restless at night.
Arnica After an injury or shock, for bruises, or before and after a visit to the dentist, for instance to help reduce bruising.
Arsen. alb. If the child is restless, has diarrhoea or is vomiting, mild food poisoning.
Belladonna If the child is hot and flushed, acute symptoms such as sore throat and headache.
Chamomilla For an irritable child who is restless. Also good also for teething and colic.
Pulsatilla If the child is weepy and fearful, needs attention and comfort.
Rhus tox. For sprains, strains and skin eruptions such as chickenpox and shingles.

Caution

Some herbal remedies have the same name as homoeopathic remedies, but are poisonous in plant form, so do not use any of the above as part of herbal remedies.

Traditional Chinese Medicine

Traditional Chinese medicine is an ancient and highly complex form of medicine. A fully qualified practitioner has had many years of study and training to enable them to correctly diagnose and treat illness. The range and mix of herbs chosen by a practitioner will be prescribed only after asking many detailed questions about your child.

It is very important always to seek the advice of a qualified practitioner. There is no regulation on the herbs that can be brought in from the Orient and many of them can be very toxic. There have been stories of patients suffering side-effects after using Chinese herbs, but this is uncommon if they are prescribed by a qualified practitioner. Used properly, they can safely produce results that conventional medicine has failed to do.

Indeed, Chinese medicine is used in NHS hospitals such as Great Ormond Street and the Royal Free in Hampstead, London.

Usage

The herbs may be given in a number of ways:

- *Decoction* Herbs are boiled whole, simmered and cooled before drinking.
- *Powder* Herbs are ground and mixed with hot water or honey.
- *Infusion* Herbs are brewed in boiling water and left to infuse. The resulting cooled solution can be drunk like a tea.
- *Pills* To be taken as recommended.
- *External application* Made as for decoction and then applied externally or given in a bath.

Useful foods to store

The following foods are always useful to have at home.
Cranberry Useful for urinary tract infections such as cystitis.

Fruit High in vitamins and antioxidants which can help protect against disease. Helpful for constipation.

Garlic Contains antiviral and antibacterial properties and can help to reduce cold symptoms such as nasal congestion. If taken regularly may help to lower blood pressure and blood cholesterol.

Ginger Chewed before and during a journey, ginger can help combat travel sickness. It is also thought to act as an expectorant for colds.

Greens Green leafy vegetables are high in vitamin C, calcium, beta carotene, folate, and iron, all of which are needed for healthy young children.

Honey Helpful for chest congestion and too much phlegm. Also thought to help heal wounds and act as a mild sedative for complaints such as sore throats, as it is thought to stimulate the body's natural painkillers, endorphins.

Lemon A natural antiseptic for minor cuts, grazes and stings. Also high in vitamin C.

Vinegar Cider vinegar in particular is thought to help problems from acne to bronchitis, eczema to sinusitis.